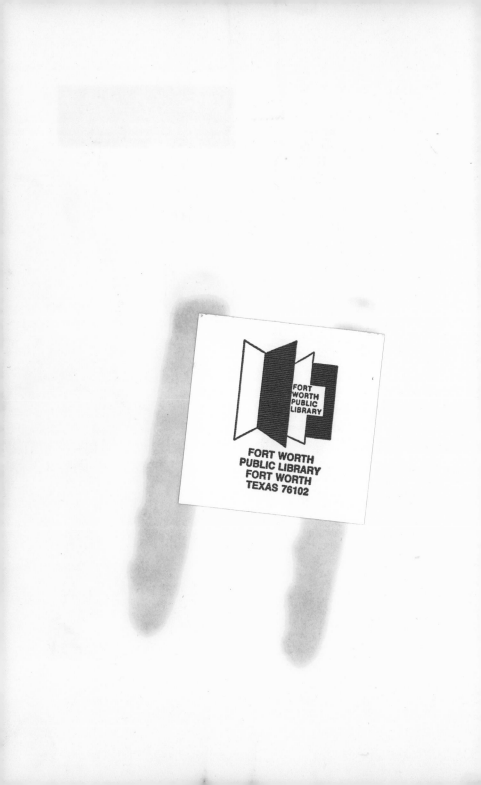

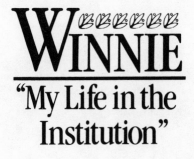

WINNIE

"My Life in the Institution"

WINNIE

"My Life in the Institution"

A Memoir of a Special Woman

by JAMIE PASTOR BOLNICK

St. Martin's/Marek
New York

Design by Doris Borowsky

Library of Congress Cataloging in Publication Data

Pastor Bolnick, Jamie.
    Winnie "My life in the institution."

    1. Sprockett, Gwynna.   2. Mentally handicapped—
United States—Biography.   3. Mentally handicapped—
Institutional care—United States—Case studies.
I. Title.
HV3006.A39S677   1985   362.3′85′0924 [B]   85-14256
ISBN 0-312-88230-0

First Edition

10 9 8 7 6 5 4 3 2 1

This book is dedicated to all the other
Winnies out there—and, especially, to
the Gwynna who might have been.

Acknowledgments

My appreciation to the superintendent of the institution where Winnie was raised, to her social worker, and to various department heads, attendants, and other workers whom I interviewed and who gave generously of their time. To preserve their privacy they shall go unnamed.

Love and special thanks to my family: to Ron for his understanding, help, and support; and to Britt and Kim, who waited "*so* long" for me to finish this project, and did it with good cheer and love. Thanks also to Pud Goodman, who first made me see the possibilities.

Most of all, my deepest gratitude to Mike McGrady, who believed when nobody else did, and gave invaluable help. Without his unflagging interest, excellent advice, and constant encouragement, Winnie's story could never have found its way onto these pages.

WINNIE'S PREFACE

The reason I wrote a book is 'cause of Willy, he's my sister's husband. He said I was mentally retarded.

"That's why you're in the institution," he told me. Right in front of my sisters, too.

"Who the hell is mentally retarded? Not me!" I hollered at him. Miriam even got mad, said, "That's a nice thing to say! Is that the way you treat someone coming to visit for Christmas?"

Willy just said, "I'm sorry that had to come out."

"Well, you didn't have to say that while she was here. You made her feel funny in front of everybody."

And when we was in the kitchen, me and Miriam and Wanda, and Miriam was doing the pies, she told me, "Don't worry about what Willy said, don't pay him no heed. Willy likes to hear hisself talk."

But I was still real mad when I got back to the institution. All I was thinking was, why did he have to go and call me that mean thing? I said to myself, "I'm gonna set down and write a book. 'Cause mentally retarded people can't write books, so I'll show Willy just how retarded I am!"

I got a notebook from Mrs. Knopf, pencils, too. It took me a long, long time to write my book. In the nights I set in the bathroom to write 'cause that's the only place they leave the lights on.

And I told everybody I was writing a book, boy, I let everyone know it. Some of the attendants, they teased me, said I thought I was a big shot 'cause I was writing a book. "Big deal, Winifred's writing a book," they said. "It's going to her head now." I didn't care.

My book proves how much I know, proves how smart I am. And anyone who reads my book is gonna say, "Who is this girl? She sure isn't mentally retarded!"

Now I'm even glad Willy called me retarded. The big mouth. He made me write that book.

ABOUT THIS BOOK

Winnie Sprockett was committed at the age of six to a state institution for mentally retarded females. She was only mildly retarded—as an adult, she had an I.Q. of about sixty-five, which roughly approximates a mental age of nine, and she acquired the equivalent of a fourth-grade education (though her reading level was higher) in the institution school.

I first knew Winnie when I was twelve years old and she was in her early twenties. My family lived less than a mile from the institution, so we often drove by it on our way into town. The institution covered several square miles of well-landscaped grounds, dotted with at least fifteen gray stone buildings. There were no bars or walls, only a big hedge that encircled most of the area. On the far side of that hedge lay a world that fascinated me. I always had the feeling when we drove by that I was glimpsing an alien race.

In the warmer months, especially, I could see the women strolling around the grounds, sitting on park benches, or sprawled casually on the grass in small, congenial-looking groups. There were always a few posted along the hedge, staring out at my world just as I was staring in at theirs. Sometimes they'd wave at the passing cars. My sister and I always waved back.

On a sunny spring Saturday when I was twelve, I leashed

up my little black dog, Gypsy, and went for a walk. Without really thinking about it, I headed for the institution. I wasn't sure why I was going there—hadn't, in fact, even realized I was when I left my house. As I got closer I considered changing directions. But I didn't.

When I approached the hedge—and it was an extremely tentative approach—two of the women spotted my dog and rushed over. Within minutes a small crowd of them had gathered to gush and flutter over Gypsy. While I held Gypsy up so they could reach over the hedge to pet and fondle her, I studied these strange creatures closely.

They weren't an attractive lot. They were all dressed in cheap house dresses, neat and clean but baggy and ill-fitting. Many had their hair cut short and square in classic institution style, though a few sported curls and ponytails. Their ages varied greatly—several didn't look much older than I, and some of the women could have been grandmothers. Lots of them were missing teeth, and some spoke in a thick, slurred speech. But they were, without a doubt, human. They talked, they laughed, they adored my dog. And that's what astonished me: these women were real people. They weren't like me or the other people I knew, but they weren't so terribly different, either. The similarities surprised me most; I'd anticipated the differences.

When the novelty of Gypsy wore off, they turned their attention to me. They admired my clothes and hair and plied me with naive questions. Where did I live? Did I like the institution? Did I like them? Did I like television? Did I have a boyfriend? They were too friendly, obsequiously friendly; they seemed frantic to establish contact. Suddenly I wanted very much to get away from them. Before I left they begged me to promise to return, and I agreed. I'd have agreed to anything just then; I wanted to go home. But I don't think, at the time, that I had any intention of returning. I'd satisfied my curiosity.

Why I went back there a couple of Saturdays later I don't remember. But I did, and after that I fell into a regular pattern of visiting. I began to learn the women's names and they came to remember mine. By my third or fourth visit, I had only to approach the hedge to draw an excited and rather flustered crowd. I loved the fuss. It made me feel like a visiting dignitary.

At first I didn't venture past the hedge. But, gradually, I became certain that I was in no danger—they would not harm me—and within a month I was sitting inside on the front lawn with the women, chatting comfortably and experiencing the exceedingly curious sensation of seeing my world from their vantage point. By early summer I knew dozens of the women, but there was a nucleus of six or seven who considered themselves my special friends, who were unabashedly possessive and sometimes, literally, hung on to me. One of these women was Winnie (though I knew her then as 'Winifred'). I have only vague memories of her from those days: a tall, ungainly young woman with short, permed hair, straight bangs, and thick eyeglasses. I do remember, though, that I enjoyed her company—I had a lot in common with Winnie and her friends. We watched the same TV shows, we liked the same movie stars, we drooled over the same rock 'n roll singers. I giggled with them about boys, laughed at their jokes, and swapped comic books with white-haired old ladies.

The women loved to talk about themselves. They all had minor beefs about institution life: some didn't like the food, others resented the nine o'clock lights-out rule. The most common complaint was that "Nobody ever comes to visit me." But I was surprised to find that most were reasonably satisfied with their lot. They were intensely interested in every little detail of my life—they were as curious about me as I was about them—but I detected no jealousy. They seemed grateful just to share the events of my life vicariously.

The women I came in contact with on those long ago Saturdays were the brighter ones, the more responsible ones, the ones who had the privilege of moving freely about the grounds. I never saw the severely retarded or disturbed women; they were kept within the confines of their buildings. In those days, the 1950s, there were many people in institutions throughout the country who, like Winnie Sprockett, were only mildly retarded. Today, most of them would have been living on the outside, independently or in group homes, perhaps holding down simple jobs. Even worse, it wasn't unusual in those days to come across an older institution resident of relatively normal intelligence who'd been committed back in the 1920s, or earlier, merely for running away from home, being caught in the hayloft with a boy, or transgressions far more minor. This institution, like many others, had originally been established for the "feeble-minded and incorrigible."

When I was thirteen we moved to another state, and the women were really sorry to say good-bye. I'd been the only visitor many of them had had for years. There were hugs and cries of, "Now don't you forget me!" and several of the ones who could read and write, including Winnie, wrote down their full names and the names of their buildings so I could write to them. I kept in touch for about half a year, and they always replied promptly in large, childish handwriting. But as I became involved with my new school and new friends, I gradually stopped writing.

Fifteen years later I saw Winnie Sprockett again. I was spending the summer in the town I'd lived in as a child and needed a temporary job. An old friend, now a psychologist at the institution I used to visit, told me that they were hiring summer help. I got a job in the Children's Cottage as one of four "recreation assistants" assigned to the children for the summer. Our function was to supervise playtime and organize games and crafts. Most of the other summer workers were graduate students in psychology and were trained to keep an emotional distance. But nothing had prepared me for children like these—the seizures, the tantrums, the way they clung to me and everyone else within clinging distance, desperate for a scrap of attention. Some days I went home and cried. I considered quitting but it was July, and I knew I'd never find another summer job. So I stuck it out.

On a sticky August day, during lunch break, I overheard a group of summer workers talking about an institution resident who'd written her autobiography. A few of them had read it. A week or so later, she came into the canteen where I was having coffee with my co-workers and they pointed her out to me. Although I hadn't yet heard her name, something clicked in my memory and I thought, instantly, "Winifred. . . ."

Fifteen years. Wonderful years for me, crammed full of living. And there was Winnie Sprockett, in exactly the same place and looking almost exactly as she had when I was thirteen. The only difference I could see was that she now wore her hair in a stubby little ponytail. It seemed absolutely incredible that we'd both lived through the same fifteen years.

She came over to say hello to the group and somebody introduced us. I didn't bother to tell her I'd known her; I was sure she'd never remember me. But I did tell her that I'd heard about her book, and I asked if I could read it.

"Could you get it published for me?" was her immediate response.

Winnie had written her book in several spurts during the early and mid-1960s. Word of it got around the institution and, in time, most of the professional staff had read it. One of the psychiatrists used it in a lecture, and it was duplicated for graduate students in social work at the state university. Suddenly Winnie, who'd been raised by state-paid attendants in an institution with 1700 other females, stood out. Winnie, who'd always craved attention, who'd always ached to be noticed, was special. She had an identity: she was "Winifred, the girl who wrote the book." And she made sure everyone knew it.

For awhile there was even talk in the institution's Psychology Department of having the book published in a psychiatric journal. The plan never materialized, but Winnie latched onto the idea and it became an obsession. She was determined to get her book published. Then it would be in bookstores and libraries, and the whole world—especially her indifferent family—would know how smart and important she was. She became a walking advertisement. She talked about the book to anyone who'd stand still long enough to listen, and was even known to approach complete strangers visiting the institution to ask if they could help her get it published. But I didn't know any of this that day in the canteen. If I had, I wouldn't have been so startled (and, I confess, a little amused) by her question.

I told Winnie that I didn't think I could get her book published, but I'd like to borrow it for a few days, anyway. She replied, agreeably, "Okay," went back to her building for the book, and I took it home with me that day.

Winnie's book was written in longhand, in pencil, in a child's black copybook. On the cover, in the space next to "Subject," she'd written the title: "My Life in the Institution." The book was short—a little more than twenty pages of large writing, divided into twenty-four choppy chapters. More than half of it dealt with her progress in the institution school, describing at great length her lessons and how hard she worked at them. She also touched on the behavior problems she'd had in her childhood and adolescence, the "troubles" she was always getting into (though she wasn't very specific about them), and gave much praise to the institution authorities for punishing her and making her behave. It seemed to me that the book was mostly intended to please and flatter the institution personnel and put a shine on Winnie's image. It was interesting simply because she'd written it, but I couldn't help wondering what she'd left out, what it had really been like for her.

A week later my job ended. I returned the book to Winnie on my last day and, early in September, I moved back to the city. Winnie and I kept in touch, though, and in her letters she frequently brought up the subject of her book, always asking if I could think of a way to get it published.

Later in the year, she was released from the institution through a social service agency and placed in a nursing home—the only available means, in those days, of moving some of the more competent inmates out into the community and, at the same time, making room in overcrowded institutions. This was Winnie's second nursing home placement; an earlier placement, detailed in this book, had failed. And so, in time, did this one.

One day I went to visit Winnie. I had with me a portable tape recorder and I showed her how it worked, let her listen to her voice, then asked if I could interview her. I wanted to know what wasn't in Winnie's book, and I wanted to try to understand how the fifteen years I'd lived so fully had passed for Winnie—or passed by Winnie.

I remained noncommittal each time Winnie talked about getting her book published. I knew the book would need a great deal of expansion; I suspected, in fact, that it could only be used as a jumping-off point for Winnie's real life story and I wasn't sure what, if anything, would develop from the interviews. But I was beginning to think about giving the project a try. I approached the whole thing tentatively, as I'd once approached the institution hedge; but very quickly, like that other time, I was drawn in.

Winnie was a perfect subject. She loved being interviewed and was talkative and animated from the start. She was nearly forty then, but she had the innocence and enthusiasms of a clever nine-year-old. She possessed an intuitive awareness of herself and other people that was almost uncanny, and a memory that was incredible. She also had a wonderful sense of the dramatic. Often, while telling me about an event, she became so caught up in it that she appeared to be reliving it rather than recalling it. She even acted out the dialogue. Frequently, especially at these times, she spoke in the present tense, as if the events were unfolding as she talked. I was completely charmed by her and, without ever really making a conscious decision, I was hooked on her story.

There were difficulties, of course. Winnie had a short attention span, so thirty minutes was about the longest I could interview her at a time, though we often did several sessions a day. She was also inconsistent. In the morning she might talk for thirty minutes with clarity, insight, and, occasionally, even eloquence. Several hours later her conversation would be disjointed; she'd be off on a tangent, not always making sense, skewing language so badly at times that I wasn't sure what she was talking about. Even at her best, she rambled a lot.

Although Winnie had a brilliant memory for dates and facts, she had a hazy sense of time in general. Incidents such as her trips out of the institution, as well as some of her escapades and adventures, were not always easy to place in time. In putting this book together, I arranged events in the order I felt was most logical and accurate. Winnie sometimes, when recalling or acting out a conversation, gave slightly different versions at different times, though the essence was always the same. Obviously, she couldn't have remembered all the actual dialogue of a lifetime, and there's no way to corroborate the exact words that were spoken in a conversation twenty or thirty years ago. I've done my best to reconstruct these conversations in the way that seemed most appropriate and corresponded most faithfully to the facts as I knew them. In a few instances I combined parts from different versions.

In order to be true to Winnie's distinctive voice, I've chosen to retain her use of the present tense throughout much of the book. For the sake of readability I've eliminated some repetitious and irrelevant material and, in several places, I've made narrative of dialogue and vice versa. All names of people (including Winnie's) and places have been changed to ensure privacy, as have certain identifying details.

During later conversations with her social worker, and lengthy interviews with institution personnel (who opened up Winnie's files for me), I was able to verify much of what

Winnie told me. Anecdotes that couldn't be verified are, nevertheless, presented here as Winnie perceived them; it was, after all, her perceptions I wanted to capture. If she sometimes recollected an event or a conversation to her own advantage, that was still Winnie's reality and therefore I considered it valid.

At the core of this book is Winnie's original book, "My Life in the Institution." But most of "Winnie" is the result of the taped interviews I conducted with her throughout that spring and summer, our many conversations, and the notes I took when we were together. Although I've arranged and edited the material in this book and chosen its form and structure, the words are Winnie's. This is Winnie's voice and Winnie's story.

One afternoon, a month or so into the interviews, Winnie and I were in a luncheonette. We'd both just polished off pieces of strawberry shortcake, her favorite treat at the time, and her upper lip was still lined with whipped cream as she started in on her root beer.

"You know, Winnie," I said, "I knew you a long time ago."

"I thought you looked familiar to me," she replied, obligingly.

"No, I'm talking about a *very* long time ago—nearly sixteen years. I used to come over to the institution to visit the girls and I remember you. You were one of the girls I used to come see."

"I remember you, too."

"It would be awfully hard for you to remember me, Winnie. I was a little girl then."

She set down her empty root beer glass and screwed up her face in hard thought.

"I sure do remember you. Didn't you use to come on a bike?"

My turn to think—I'd had a blue Schwinn and, yes, I'd often ridden over to the institution on it. I'd forgotten that.

"And didn't you sometimes bring a littler girl with you?"

Another thing I'd forgotten: sometimes my younger sister had come along.

"You're right, Winnie," I told her, "on both counts."

Perhaps other neighborhood youngsters had visited the women, too; perhaps she was confusing me with someone from a more recent time. Or maybe she really did remember.

She licked the rest of the whipped cream from her lip and beamed at me. "Well, I sure am glad to see you again!" she said.

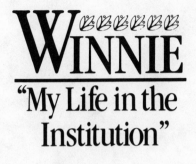

WINNIE
"My Life in the Institution"

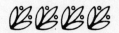

SUMMER
1938

1

God give me a good memory. I can remember that day real well. My mother was giving me a bath and telling me I was going away. But she wouldn't tell me where, just that I was going for a long ride in the car. I was six years old.

She dressed me in my prettiest dress, red with yellow flowers. It had a rip under the arm 'cause it belonged to my sister Wanda first, but always I kept my arm down whenever I wore that dress so no one could see the hole. I liked that dress, it made me feel pretty like Wanda.

It started to rain and thunderstorm and the wipers, the windshield wipers, didn't work too good. My mother kept saying bad words and she had to drive real slow; we drove and drove a long time. I set in back. And she didn't talk to me, she never liked to talk to me, she never even loved me. Maybe that's 'cause she wasn't my real mother. So I just set there, and sometimes I wondered where we was going 'cause we never drove so far away before, and sometimes I tried to look out the window. But I couldn't always see good—too much rain.

Then I started feeling like I needed to go to the bathroom, and I had to tell my mother, and she had to look for a gas station so I could go. I got all wet running into that bathroom, even my shoes got wet. My mother waited in the car, she didn't want to get wet. We drove some more and pretty soon I had to go again. I tried to set real still to hold it, I tried crossing my legs on the seat of the car, but still I had to go. My mother got real mad 'cause she had to find another gas station. But I couldn't help it, that's how I always do when I'm nervous.

I was getting hungry, too, and my stomach was starting up to make growly noises, but I didn't think I better say anything about that.

2

We went through some big gates, we drove up a driveway. I seen lots of gray buildings—big gray buildings and little gray buildings. I thought, "Hmmmmm, what's this place?" and I was glad to get out of that darn car 'cause I sure was tired of setting there.

I got all wet running from the parking lot, my mother got all wet, too. We went into a building full of offices. There was people setting behind desks and some was writing stuff and some was talking on the phone in a busy way. My mother took me up to a lady who was setting at one of them desks. She said, "This here's Winnie Sprockett."

I didn't want to meet the lady, I didn't want to leave go my mother's hand, didn't even know what I was doing in that place. The lady told me to come with her.

"But I'm all wet," I said.

My mother told me, "You go with her, Winnie, and I'm gonna wait right here 'cause you'll be back soon."

The lady took me to another building. We had to walk up some long driveways past a whole bunch of other buildings, but at least she had an umbrella. Inside the building I seen nurses, lots of nurses.

I ask, "Is this a hospital?" My daddy was in a hospital once. The lady said yes, it was a hospital.

I told her I wasn't sick but she wouldn't listen, or could be she couldn't understand me 'cause my speech wasn't too good. A nurse took off my wet clothes and she made me wear a funny little nightie that didn't close up all the way, and then I started to cry. I said, "But I'm not sick, I'm just wet, even my shoes is wet, but I'm gonna dry off soon!"

I wanted my red dress with the flowers back, I wanted my mother. I knew my mother didn't even love me, but when they put that funny nightie on me, I wanted her. I was so scared I wasn't even hungry no more. I told them my mother was waiting on me in the office and she was gonna be mad if I took too long. I cried, I screamed, I yelled. They just kept telling me, "Calm down, Winifred. You got to calm down."

"No! I wanna go back to my mother!"

But they didn't pay me no mind. Just carried me to a big room with beds, and got people in the beds, all the while I was kicking and screaming. I thought they was stealing me. They tried to put me down and I jump out of the bed and they tried to put me down and up I pop again.

Then they give me a shot—boy, two nurses had to hold me so they could stick that thing in my arm. I slept for a long time, even though it wasn't my bedtime.

When I woke up, the people in the other beds was sleeping. Outside the window was dark. I thought, maybe my mother got tired of setting and waiting in that office until it got to be dark, maybe she drove home without me and left me all alone in this place. I cried so hard the slobber come all down my nightie. The girl in the next bed said, "Shut up!" so I jump out of bed and start hitting on her. Right away a nurse come running, grab me, she push me back on my bed.

"I want my mother, I want my mother!" I yelled.

Another nurse come too, they set with me on my bed holding me, they was saying things like, "Hush, hush, Winifred, you woke everybody up." But I didn't give a darn who I woke up. They had some juice, they told me when I be calm I could have a drink. I did want a drink, my throat was hurting me from all the yelling I done that day. I drunk up all the juice in the cup. When I was done, one of the nurses said, "Your mother had to go home, it was getting late. You go to sleep now, then your mother's gonna come back real soon."

I laid back down, I put the pillow over my head so they couldn't hear me crying. I missed my mother so much. She never give me no loving, but still I missed her. And I missed my daddy. He wasn't my real daddy, neither, but that didn't bother him, he was good to me. I helped him with the chickens. All the time he said to me, "Oh, Winnie, you're a real big help with the chickens." That did make me feel so proud.

I didn't miss my sisters much, only Gladys; I never got along too good with Wanda and Miriam. And Wanda was all the time picking on me. Most of all I missed Patches. He always slept on my bed with me and you could say I wasn't use to being in bed without Patches.

By the time morning come, my whole pillow was all over wet.

Them other people woke up, I could see in the light they was girls and ladies. There wasn't a lot, and most was grown-up, except for the kid in the next bed I hit.

The nurses give me my breakfast, brung it to me in bed. They said, "Are you gonna behave today?" I said yes. I was feeling too tired to fuss much about anything.

All day they done tests on me, healthy tests, see if I'm healthy or not healthy. They stuck a needle in my arm and took my blood away from me, but I didn't even cry. They told me to go to the bathroom in a paper cup, they took X-ray pictures of me.

They done talking tests, too. Like the doctor ask me stuff, mostly stuff I didn't know, like my numbers and letters and how to spell my name and how many fingers I got on my hands. Whatever I said he wrote down with a pencil, even when I said, "I don't know," he wrote that down. Also he ask me to look at pictures and play games, such as blocks.

Then the doctor wanted to talk about my mother and daddy. Not the mother and daddy I got that the State give me, the real mother and daddy that died. He wanted to know if I did remember them or if I didn't remember them. But I just said, "I don't know," again 'cause I don't always like to talk about that. So we talked about my sisters. I told him they are Gladys, Miriam, and Wanda. They are my real sisters, I didn't get them from the State. I had them already.

All the day I tried to be nice. I wanted to be good so they wouldn't be mad. I thought maybe if I was good, my mother would come sooner and take me home. When they took me back to the hospital room with all them beds I said, "But when is my mother coming? Isn't my mother coming?"

They told me, "Your mother isn't coming today, have some supper," and they brung me my supper, but I wouldn't eat. I was good all day and my mother didn't come, so I had enough of trying to be good. I kicked my tray, my supper tray, and it fell off the bed. There was noodles all over the place. Boy, was I dumb, I was dumb as a doornail, 'cause I was still waiting for my mother to come and get me. It's a good thing I didn't know she wasn't coming, I would of broke everything in the place.

Some more nurses come, they held me down, give me another shot. They sure liked to give people shots in that place. I never did get more supper 'cause then I went to sleep, slept all the night long.

3

First thing I seen when I woke up in the morning time was my red dress with the yellow flowers. It was laying on my bed. Did I ever set up fast. I thought it must be that I was going home, must be that my mother come back to the office. I wanted to take off my funny nightie and put that dress on quick. Trouble was, I didn't know how to dress myself. But I was so happy. I was sick of that place. I wondered, did Patches miss me?

A nurse come and dressed me. They didn't have my socks, said they got lost, but I didn't care if I had to put my shoes on with no socks. My feets felt funny in my shoes with no socks, but that was okay by me.

The nurse was real nice. The kind of nurse that likes you. She took me downstairs and there was this big lady waiting for me. She had a white dress on, too, like a nurse's dress, but no cap.

"This here's Winifred," the nurse told the big lady, and she told me the big lady was Mrs. Spencer. Mrs. Spencer didn't smile at all, she didn't have a nice look. She had an old face. She took ahold of my hand and I ask her, "Are we going to the office? Is my mother at the office?" I don't know if she could understand me, or maybe she just didn't want to talk. We started walking.

We walked and walked and I seen lots of ladies outside by the gray buildings. Some was walking and some was setting. I even seen some ladies swinging on swings. I thought that was funny. I never seen grown-up ladies swinging before. Only thing, they all got short hair, they all got short hair almost like a boy's hair. And strange dresses, ugly dresses. I also seen ladies in white dresses like Mrs. Spencer. They got hair like regular.

It was real hot and I was getting tired of walking, going

slower and slower, and Mrs. Spencer had to tell me to
hurry up. Then we come to this building, it was little and
got bars on all the windows like cages. I stopped to look.
Could be they got animals in there. But it wasn't animals, it
was faces, I seen faces peeping out the bars at me. They got
people in there.

"Come on, Winifred!" Mrs. Spencer said.

"What are them people doing?"

Then I heard a terrible scream come from that building. It
sounded like nothing you ever want to remember. Boy, did
I go fast, Mrs. Spencer didn't have to tell me to hurry up. I
didn't like that place, didn't like the funny ladies they got
there, didn't like that scary building with the screaming
coming out.

I ask Mrs. Spencer, "Where is my mother? Where is that
office?"

"We're not going to the office, we're going to the Children's Cottage."

"No, I wanna go home now!" But she didn't say nothing
else.

The building she took me to was gray like the other
buildings, but it was littler, it looked like a house almost.
And got a yard with a fence and little swings and a sandbox
and all stuff like that. We went up the steps and she took me
into a little room, got a lady in there setting at a desk. Mrs.
Spencer had some papers from the nurse at the hospital, and
she give the papers to the lady. She said, "This here's
Winifred." The lady, who was Mrs. Treadwell, put on her
glasses and looked at the papers. Then she took off her
glasses, said, "Okay, give her to Mrs. Drake."

Mrs. Spencer took me down a long hall and I seen these
kids lined up, big girls and little girls. They was all in their
nighties and making lots of noises. Some of them was kind
of peculiar looking, too. Mrs. Spencer said, "Bath time,"
and she give me to a colored lady in a white dress. Told the
lady, "This here's Winifred Sprockett and she's a new kid."

The colored lady told me to go in line to get my bath. I

said, "I don't want no bath. I don't want to stay here." Mrs. Spencer pushed me into the line.

It was such a funny bathroom, I never seen such a bathroom like they got there. Lots of little toilets and lots of little sinks in that bathroom, and three bathtubs. You stand in line for your bath, and there was even two lines, one for kids in wheeling chairs. I was wondering why them kids got to set down and the other kids had to stand up.

I didn't want to get my dress took off when it come my turn, didn't want to get it took off in front of all them people. You could say I wasn't use to it, I was shy, didn't know nobody. The colored lady, Mrs. Drake, she talked to me nice. She wasn't old and grumpy like Mrs. Spencer. So I let her take off my clothes, but still I felt shy. She put me in the tub, she washed me. I didn't like it. The water got hair in it and it wasn't too warm, it was mostly cold. They was using the same water for all the kids.

After I got my bath, Mrs. Drake put my red dress back on me, she give me some socks and clean bloomers, she tie my shoes. Someone brushed my teeths for me at one of them funny little sinks—I couldn't even brush my teeths then. At home Miriam always brushed my teeths for me, dressed me, too.

Mrs. Drake said I could go get my breakfast and she told another kid to take me, she told the kid that was Ruby Rose to take me. She was the only kid real little like me, the other kids was bigger than me. She took me to the basement and that was where the dining room and the playroom was. Kids was setting at long tables eating. They sure was funny kids. A couple of them got heads which looked too big, or teeths poking out; a couple was shaped wrong in the body. And they knew how to be noisy, too, made so much noise talking and yelling to each other and eat real messy. Food on their faces. Some was trying to eat with their fingers, thought it was funny to eat cereal with their fingers, or maybe they just didn't know no better. I never seen kids doing like that before, never seen kids acting up like that.

I set next to Ruby Rose, ate all my breakfast, every bit, but I was still hungry. They didn't give me enough. "I want more cereal, I want more applesauce," I told the lady.

She said, "So does all the other kids."

I didn't think it was fair that you couldn't get seconds. I got a big appetite.

After breakfast, when all the kids went out to that little yard, Mrs. Spencer come to get me. I thought I was going home. But she took me up to the bathroom, she got a chair, she got big scissors, she told me, "Set down."

"What are you gonna do?"

"Cut your hair."

"Cut my hair?" Miriam always made me braids. I had real long hair. Sometimes, when Miriam was being nice to me, or for special, she even put ribbons in my braids. I liked my braids, I liked how they jumped when I jumped.

I told Mrs. Spencer, "Maybe my mother might be mad. Maybe my mother don't want me to get my hair cut." But she just combed my hair and started cutting. She cut and cut and cut, and my hair fell down all over me and all over the floor. I thought she wasn't gonna leave me nothing on my head at all.

When she was done, I put up my hands to feel. I could feel my ears sticking out, that's how short she cut my hair. Short like them other kids and ladies.

I told Mrs. Spencer, "I don't think my mother's gonna like my hair the way you cut it." But she act like she didn't care if my mother didn't like it, didn't even give a darn if my mother might be mad. I started to cry.

Mrs. Spencer told me to go out in the yard, but I didn't want to. I was all worked up, and anyway I was ashamed. I knew I looked funny with my ears sticking out. My ears was never sticking out before. I ask Mrs. Spencer, "When is my mother coming?" but she couldn't understand me with all that crying, or maybe she could understand me but she didn't want to tell me. Maybe she knew I'd never stop crying if she told me my mother wasn't coming.

A big girl took me out to the yard and I set there in a corner of the sandbox all by myself, crying. I tried to cover my ears with my hands, tried not to look at them other kids, but I couldn't help it. Some was playing on the swings and seesaw but some wasn't playing, just stood there and rocked or shook their hands in front of their face. One was singing. They looked to me to be real dumb. And when they move or walk they go all jerky. It was strange, it sure looked strange to me. I never seen such kinds of kids before. They even scared me a little bit 'cause I wasn't use to kids which was peculiar like that.

I kept wondering, why did my mother ever bring me to this place, anyway? What was this kind of place? Why did she go home and leave me here? Must be she didn't know they got peculiar kinds of kids here, or maybe no one told her.

Ruby Rose come over with another girl. They stood there, watched me crying and covering my ears. That got me so mad I hollered bad words and threw sand. Then the bigger girls come and start to laugh at me. They was telling each other stuff like, "Look at little new girl, setting there crying."

"So what. I could cry if I want to."

And this big fat girl, the big fat girl that was Estelle Sampson—she was one of the kids with them big heads— she threw sand at me. So I had to throw sand back at her. And I told her, "My mother is coming soon and taking me home. I'm not staying in this place!"

"She thinks she's going home," Estelle Sampson said. "She's so dumb she thinks she's going home." And she told me, "You're not going home, you're gonna stay here forever!"

"That's what you think! I'm going home right now!"

And I run right out of that yard.

I was gonna find that office place all by myself. Maybe

my mother come back, maybe my mother was waiting in the office a long time and no one would tell her where I was. So many buildings. How could she tell wherever did they put me? I start running up one of the driveways. My hair felt funny when I run, no braids left to bump up and down.

I heard Mrs. Spencer yelling, "Winifred! Winifred!" She was coming after me. I didn't want her to catch me, I had to find the office before my mother got tired of waiting and went home without me again. Then she might never come back. It took such a long time to drive here and my mother didn't like to drive a lot. I called, "Mommy! Mommy! Mommy!" and run fast as I could, turned up another driveway, and then Mrs. Spencer wasn't behind me no more.

There was ladies setting on a bench, got short hair and them dresses. They laughed and yelled, "Where you going, little girl?" But I didn't stop. I was getting real hot and my feets hurt 'cause my shoes was a little small, but I kept running. There was buildings all over the place, but I didn't see none that looked like the office. And every time I pass some of them ladies with their funny dresses, they call out to me and laugh. All the way up that driveway I run, all the way until I got to the end where there was only just fields. No office. Wrong driveway.

I start going back and then I seen Mrs. Spencer again, only this time she was coming at me with two other ladies in white dresses. They was yelling at me to stop. I didn't know where to go—they was coming at me too fast—so I run real quick around this big building. I could hear noises, like howling, behind the building. Noises like Patches makes when he howls 'cause there's a rabbit outside, or he wants to come in and my mother won't let him. I thought there was a dog back there. But when I got around to the back of the building, I seen it wasn't no dog at all, it was a lady. A lady setting in a wheeling chair on the grass. She was a grown-up, but she was wearing a baby bib and a shirt and big diapers. Her mouth was open and that noise, that howl noise like Patches makes, was coming out. And her diaper, her great big diaper, was bloody.

I stopped and I stood there and I screamed. I was afraid to keep going and I was afraid of Mrs. Spencer coming after me the other way. I didn't know what to do, where to go, and my legs wouldn't move no more, had to set down real quick on the grass. I was hot and sweaty, but I was shivering, too.

When Mrs. Spencer and them other ladies catched me, Mrs. Spencer pulled me up and she shook me and shook me until I thought I was gonna throw up all over Wanda's dress. Boy, was she ever mad 'cause I made her run so far. Her face was all sweaty and red. She told the other ladies, "This kid is a real trouble maker. Hold her tight so she don't get away again." Mrs. Spencer and one of the ladies grabbed my arms hard, they hurt me. But they didn't need to do that. I wasn't going nowhere. I couldn't run no more 'cause my legs quit on me, and anyway what could I do? I was little, they was big. All I wanted was to get away from that lady, the lady with the blood and noises.

They took me back to the kids' building and always they kept pulling my arms. Once I almost fell down 'cause my legs wouldn't go right, but they was holding me so tight I couldn't fall. When they got me back, they took me to the big room where all the beds was and they took off my clothes. They put a nightie on me, it felt scratchy but at least it closed up all the way, and Mrs. Drake come in with medicine in a spoon and she made me take it. I laid in my bed real quiet, laid there a long time. I didn't even cry.

4

Oh, the nighttime was awful. In the big room for sleeping there was lots of beds, lots of kids, and after Miss Busby turned off the lights, was there ever lots of noises. The girls screamed in their sleep, the girls called for their mommys, sometimes they banged their heads. I didn't know what the heck was going on, it frightened me to lay in the dark and listen to all that stuff. The bed was hard, too, not soft and comfy like at home.

Then I start to go to sleep and I heard this most terrible noise. I set up real quick in bed. One of the girls was on the floor, she was rolling and screaming and making animal kind of noises. Miss Busby and the other ladies turned on the lights and run in. They had to hold her down on the floor, then they had to give her some medicine. In awhile she got calm down again.

Ruby Rose was in the next bed to me. I ask her, "Why is that girl on the floor?"

She told me, "She got the fits."

Another kid got the fits that night, too. And I'd have to wake up, you can't sleep with all that going on. Miss Busby give her the calm medicine and she went back to sleep, but I couldn't. I just laid there, didn't want to go back to sleep 'cause I didn't know if someone else was gonna get the fits and wake me up and scare me all over again. I wasn't use to it. Too many kids, too much noises, fits, fits, fits. At home I only had to sleep with Wanda and Miriam, and they didn't have the fits, they didn't make noises. At home Patches was always on my bed. At home was quiet, quiet and still for sleeping.

I laid there and I start thinking about what Estelle Sampson said, that I wasn't never going home. Maybe she just liked to see me cry. Or maybe what she said could even be true. If I was going home, why was I still here? Why didn't my mother come and get me already? She should of took me home when the hospital said I'm healthy. But she didn't.

Could be she left me here 'cause I wasn't a good girl. Always in the trouble, any trouble I could find I get right into it. Like taking money from her pocketbook when she told me I better not do that again, or breaking her watch, or socking Wanda when I got real mad and had a tamper. Maybe she left me here 'cause I was always carrying on and throwing tampers, maybe she just didn't want a kid who done them things. Or maybe she left me here 'cause I was a nervous girl, I wasn't a normal girl like Wanda and Miriam and Gladys. My nerves is bad, their nerves is good.

But even if my mother didn't want me, I knew my daddy wanted me.

So then I got to thinking, well, maybe my daddy don't know where she took me. How could he? He didn't come with us. But I bet as soon as he finds out where she took me, he's gonna come get me. 'Cause I help him so much with the chickens. Who's gonna help him with the chickens if I'm not there? Not Wanda.

Then I felt better. I thought I just had to wait for my daddy to come get me. It was taking a long time, but I just had to wait. I thought about me and Patches running through the woods behind the chicken coops, I thought about the chickens coming out clucking and making happy noises, all excited to see me back home. That helped me to go to sleep. I didn't hear no more fits that night.

When I woke up I wasn't feeling so bad.

Mrs. Drake put a different dress on me. I ask her where was mine, she said it was being washed. I didn't like this dress. It was blue and it didn't fit me too good.

After we got our breakfast, we went out in the yard. I didn't want to go, I wanted to stay inside, I was afraid Estelle Sampson and them others was gonna bother me. But you have to go, you can't say you don't want to, you gotta do like they say. So I set in the corner of the sandbox again. Only this time I wasn't crying and could be that's why I didn't get teased.

There was some toys out there. A busted baby buggy and a tricycle. Ruby Rose was riding the tricycle, she could sure go fast. I never rode a tricycle before. I wanted to do it, go fast like Ruby Rose, but I was too shy to try.

While I was setting in the sandbox, I heard a "quack-quack" and I spied a duck, a real live duck. It was walking around near the yard. I hollered, "Look, look, a duck!" and Mrs. Treadwell—she was in the yard talking to Mrs. Spencer—she opened the gate and let the duck come into the yard. She said it lived near the building and come to play with the kids all the time, said his name was Donald Duck. I went "quack-quack" at him and he went "quack-quack" back at me. He was real friendly. I liked him, I liked him better than the kids. I knew he wasn't gonna tease me. When it come to be lunch time, I didn't even want to go in to get my lunch, didn't want to leave Donald Duck.

After lunch Donald Duck wasn't there. I looked and called and I even go "quack-quack," but no Donald Duck. Then I thought maybe I could try to ride that tricycle. I didn't know if I could make it go, but I really did want to learn it. When my daddy come there I'd be, riding that tricycle all over the darn place, and wouldn't his eyes just pop out.

But when I set on the tricycle, Ruby Rose come over to get it back. She pulled the tricycle, so I had to get off and pull it too, keep her from getting it away from me. I give a hard pull, and Ruby Rose fell right on top of the tricycle, bumped her face. She set up such a yell. Mrs. Spencer come running, started hollering at me. And Ruby Rose got to ride the tricycle. I wanted to sock her.

I had trouble sleeping again that night. More noises, more fits. And every time a kid gets a fit the ladies come in, turn on the lights, got to quiet the kid and give her the calm medicine. That made the kid go back to sleep, but it didn't do nothing for me. I just laid there and laid there.

Always in my thoughts was home. Like I wondered, where was Patches sleeping? Was he sleeping on my bed still? Maybe he started sleeping on Wanda's bed. That got me mad, to think that.

So I thought about the chickens, how I get the eggs and Patches comes with me. I put the eggs in a big basket when I get them, I carry the basket real careful so as not to break the eggs. My best job is feeding the chickens. Chickens are soft when they are little and I hold them in my hands to get the softness of them. I laid there in my bed and thought of the softness of little chickies in my hands. I laid there in my bed and thought about all them things while I waited for the next fits to come.

I didn't get a whole lot of sleep.

5

In the morning all the kids was in a dither. They was talking and buzzing about visiting day. Mabel said, "My mommy's coming to see me and she's bringing me lots of chocolate candy."

"Who cares?" Estelle Sampson told her. "When my mommy and daddy come they is bringing me chocolate candy and chocolate cake and chocolate cookies."

All the girls was getting their baths, getting dressed, eating breakfast, all the girls was talking, talking, talking, about who was coming to see them and what goodies they was gonna get. I got real excited. I thought it must be the day my mother and daddy was coming. And when my daddy seen me he'd take me right away home, no matter what my mother said.

Mrs. Spencer give me another dress to wear. It was stripey yellow and green and it was big, bigger than the blue one yesterday. Come almost down to the bottom of my legs. I must of looked awful funny in that ugly dress and got all my hair cut off. What was my mother and daddy gonna say when they seen me?

After we got our breakfast, we had to go out to the yard, and in a little while Mrs. Spencer come to get Josephine 'cause her mother was there, then she come to get Lucy. We seen Josephine riding down the driveway in a big car, then we seen Lucy going, too.

The kids in the yard, the dumb ones, they was rocking and singing and playing with their hands like always. Like they didn't know nothing, like they didn't care what was going on. But the other ones was all waiting, not even playing, just standing by the fence watching the driveway to see who was coming. So was I doing that, my mother had an old black car and I kept looking for that car. I seen some cars go by, even seen an old black car like my mother got, but it went to another building, didn't come to our building, and the people who got out weren't my mother and daddy. Wrong car.

The kids was talking about the stuff they was gonna get when their families come, and they kept waiting and waiting. Finally Mrs. Spencer come out again. She called Ruby Rose.

Donald Duck come quacking by, he wanted to get into the yard. But I didn't have no time for him, didn't care to play. I was waiting too hard.

Lunchtime. Some of the kids started getting grouchy.

"See, your mommy isn't coming and you're not getting no chocolate candy, neither," Estelle Sampson told Mabel.

Mabel yelled, "Well, least my mommy comes sometimes. No one ever come to see you."

Estelle Sampson hit Mabel, hit her right in the face, give her a bloody nose. Mabel couldn't do much about it on account of she was in a wheeling chair, her legs didn't go at all. She just set there and screamed, "Mrs. Spencer! Mrs. Drake!" and one of the kids run in to tell that Mabel got a bloody nose. She got a bloody dress, too, by the time someone come. They had to put ice on Mabel, and Estelle Sampson had to stay in the rest of the whole day long, didn't get no lunch, no dinner, neither. Served her right.

Even after it was lunchtime, I was thinking my mother and daddy was coming. I knew I was very far away, I knew they had to drive a long time to get here. That could make them be late. I set in the yard all afternoon and looked for the car.

The other girls was all nasty by then 'cause they didn't get no visitors. They was grumping and growling and being mean to anyone that talked to them or even come near. Minnie told one of the littler kids, the kid that was Edith, that her mother wasn't coming to see her 'cause she was too dumb. That made Edith cry. And when Mrs. Drake hollered at Minnie, she got the fits right there in the yard in the daytime. They had to carry her inside, she was kicking and screaming and making them awful noises. Wet her pants, too.

It was a terrible afternoon. But I kept waiting. Stood by the fence, and when I get tired from standing I go set on a swing for awhile, then go back to the fence again. I could tell when it got near to supper time. I could smell the supper smells coming out to the yard. Ruby Rose come back with her mother and she had a big doll, the kind with yellow curls. It was brand new. She said, "Look, look!" and some of the kids run over to see that doll, it was so pretty, but some of them didn't want to. They was feeling too bad.

When it come time for supper I told Mrs. Drake, "I can't go in, I gotta wait here for my mother and daddy." I wanted to stay in the yard so my mother and daddy could see me, so they could find me. If they didn't see me out there, how was they gonna know where I was?

Mrs. Drake told me, "Looks like they're not coming today."

"Yes, they are."

"You got to go get your supper now, Winifred, and maybe next week your mother and daddy is gonna come." Then she went to get Edith, make her come in for supper. Edith was still out there waiting, too.

Ruby Rose was making believe her doll was real, making believe to give it food, and wiped off the doll's mouth with her napkin. That doll even got teeths, and a big smile, and all them curls of hair. I didn't like it that she had that doll, and that her mother come, and no one come to take me home, no one give me nothing. I never even had a doll before. I set there watching Ruby Rose feed that pretty doll. It made me feel mad, it did. So I smacked her.

"Mrs. Spencer, Mrs. Spencer!" Ruby Rose yelled, "Winifred hit me!" And she start to bang me on the head with the doll, banging and banging my head. It hurt, that doll hurt me. I had to pull it away and throw it on the floor, get it all busted, so she couldn't hit me with it no more.

Mrs. Spencer come running, she said, "I had enough of that kid. I had enough of Winifred!" Ruby Rose was crying real hard and the other kids was all looking at her doll on the floor. It was busted in the head and the dress was tore, the pretty red and white dress. Mrs. Spencer grab me and carried me to the bathroom. All the way up I was yelling, "I can't help it, Ruby Rose hit me with that doll, don't get mad at me!" I was scared of Mrs. Spencer. Even when she was just standing there Mrs. Spencer had a mean look on. I bet she had a mean look when she was sleeping.

She got me in a corner of the bathroom and started smacking, not just my backside but my front side, too, kept turning me around to hit new spots. She smacked and smacked and I yowled and yowled. By the time she was done, she was huffing and puffing. Even my mother never smacked me so long. She pulled me into the bedroom, she pushed me onto my bed, she stomp out. I just laid there and cried. I was doing a lot of crying in that place.

I got up once to look out the window 'cause there was another old black car going by, but it didn't stop.

When we was all going to bed Josephine and Lucy was telling what they done with their families. They both went to town and got their supper in restaurants. They didn't have no goodies, no candy or cake or cookies, but they had real happy looks.

AUTUMN
1939

6

Mrs. Drake learned me how to ride the tricycle. She showed me where to put my feets, she showed me where to put my hands, she told me to push and push with my feets. It was hard, but I worked and worked a long time to do my legs just right, and at last I could make the tricycle go. I had trouble with the steering part, though. Couldn't remember to push my legs and turn the handle the right way all at the same time. I kept getting mixed up, got so mixed up I fell right off the tricycle. I didn't hurt myself, just got my hands and knees all dirty. Every day I would try, and finally I got so I could do it, steer that tricycle anyplace I wanted to. Then round and round the yard I go, faster and faster and faster I go. No one could catch me when I'm going like that.

I was learning other things, too. Learned to brush my teeths. Mrs. Drake showed me how to hold the toothbrush the right way, she showed me to put the powder on the toothbrush without getting it on the floor too much, showed me to rub my teeths hard to get them all cleaned. Then one day I done it all by myself, didn't need no help. I liked to brush, I liked to do things by myself.

Also learned to put my dress and bloomers on. You got to lay them down first, figure out which is the back and which is the front. Lots of the times I put my dress on the wrong way, then someone had to turn it around on me.

I couldn't button, though, that was too hard. One of the attendants or the bigger girls had to button me. Also couldn't tie my shoelaces; that was the hardest thing of all.

It felt good to brush my teeths, it felt good to put on my clothes. It made me feel like I was growing up. Like I was getting smarter.

The pretty lady was going back and forth in the driveway; she was pushing a little girl in a wheeling chair. I never seen such a pretty lady. I stood by the fence just looking at her. She got on a dress that was all over flowers and got blonde hair. Sure didn't look like no attendant to me. And the little girl was pretty, too, pretty like the lady.

The lady waved at me, she seen me looking. I felt shy, but I waved back anyway. Next time she come by she said, "Hello, what's your name?"

I ask her, "Is that your little girl?"

"Yes, this here's my little girl. Her name is Jeannie."

The little girl got blonde hair too, just like her mother. I wished I had a mother like that, a pretty friendly mother with smiles on the face.

Next visiting day there she was again, pushing Jeannie up and down the driveway in the wheeling chair. She got on another dress even prettier than the flower dress. She was smiling and singing to Jeannie and Jeannie was waving her little arms and laughing, act just like a baby. But she wasn't a baby. You could tell, you could tell she was nearly as old as me.

Jeannie's mother seen me watching and she come over to the yard and said hello again.

"Where does Jeannie live?"

"Right over there. Forest Building," she told me. Forest Building was next to us. It was for low-grades.

"You got a pretty dress."

Jeannie's mother give me a big smile, said, "Thank you." Very smiley lady.

7

"Winifred, you and Ruby Rose is gonna start school tomorrow," Mrs. Drake told me. "Teacher says it's time 'cause you're almost eight years old."

"I don't want to go to school," I said. "School is too hard. I rather stay here and play."

A lot of kids went to school. Not the real retarded ones that don't know what they're doing, that rock back and forth and got baby ways of theirselves—not them. But the smart girls, the ones that could talk a lot, they went to school. Estelle Sampson and Josephine and Lucy and Bettyann and Edith and Helen. Even the girls in wheeling chairs went. Every morning after breakfast time, Mrs. Spencer or Mrs. Drake took them kids to school. It wasn't near the Children's Cottage, it was up another driveway. Then at lunchtime they bring them kids back.

Just me and Ruby Rose was left with the retarded kids, and sometimes Minnie. She couldn't always go to school, too much fits. I didn't like staying with the retarded kids, but I didn't want to go to school, neither. Had too much school at my mother's house. I couldn't do the things the other kids could do when I went to school by my mother's house. Couldn't do my alphabet or remember my letters and numbers or spell my name. Couldn't even hold a pencil right. And the other kids teased me, too, called me "Winnie-the-Ninny." Maybe they thought I wasn't smart, or maybe they called me that 'cause they couldn't always understand me when I talked. I felt ashamed at school. I felt different from the other kids.

So I didn't care if I had to stay in the yard when the other girls went to school. I could play with Donald Duck, I could ride the tricycle whenever I got it away from Ruby Rose. I learned to do tumbersaults on the rings that was hanging from the swings. I could dig in the sandbox. Didn't bother me none.

"This school isn't gonna be too hard," Mrs. Drake told me. "It's a special kind of school, you're gonna learn lots. Maybe you could even learn to read in books."

Reading. Well, that sounded good. I could set there and instead of looking at the pictures, I could find out what the books was saying. I could read stories. Gladys use to read me stories, and sometimes Miriam use to tell me stories when she was being nice to me. If I could learn to read, the books could tell me stories. I could do stories whenever I wanted to. I thought that might be such fun. I wanted to learn to read.

So the next morning, when all the girls got took to school, Ruby Rose and me got took, too. I felt nervous. But I couldn't wait to read.

We all set in one room in the schoolhouse, big and little girls. Right away I liked the teacher, I seen her and right away I sure did like her. You could say she had a friendly look. She looked at me with a nice face. Looked like she liked me.

"Hello, Winifred. Hello, Ruby Rose. I'm Mrs. Knopf. I'm so glad I got you in my class." When people talk to you like that, look at you friendly, it makes you feel real good.

She told me and Ruby Rose to set next to each other. I had a desk, a real desk, just for me. I felt so important! The desk opened and shut and got some pencils and papers inside. For me to use. Also crayons, but some of them was broke.

First Mrs. Knopf told me and Ruby Rose to draw some pictures while the big girls was doing their work. I tried to draw with the crayons, but it was hard. I wasn't use to drawing. Never learned how. So I made scribbles with all the different colors and I kept thinking, well, when am I gonna learn to read in books?

Mrs. Knopf told me, "You gotta learn your letters and numbers first, Winifred." She showed me how to make some letters, such as A, B, and C, and she made me write them over and over. I got tired of writing them and I wasn't doing it too good, anyway, couldn't make my letters look like her letters. So she had to show me how to use the pencil right, I wasn't holding the pencil the right way.

All I done the first morning was color with crayons and try to make some letters. When it come time to go back to the building I said, "But when am I gonna learn to read?"

Mrs. Knopf patted me on my head. I liked that. She said, "You're gonna learn to read, Winifred. It just takes a long time and you gotta work real hard. But I know you're gonna learn 'cause you're a smart girl."

That made me feel so good, that she said I was a smart girl. 'Cause all the kids is always calling you dumb or retarded. Nobody ever called me a smart girl before. I liked Mrs. Knopf so much. You could say I liked the way she talked to me.

Every time we walk to school, we have to pass that funny building, the one with bars on the windows. Always you could see faces peeping out the bars, ladies' faces. But the worse thing was the screaming and yelling. Sometimes the ladies would yell words at us, terrible nasty words. Or else they would be screaming, someone screaming like they was dying.

"That's the jail," Helen told me. "It's a jail for the bad ladies, the ones that do bad."

Estelle Sampson said, "That's where Winifred's gonna get put if she don't act good. They stick pins in your behind. They kill you."

I didn't know if that was true or not true. Estelle Sampson liked to make other kids get scared. But whenever we come by that place, that jail—it was called the Behavior Center—I run like heck. Try to get past real quick so I don't have to see them ladies in the bars, so I don't have to hear all them screams.

Could be what Estelle Sampson said wasn't true, could be what she said was true. They must do something awful to them ladies to make them yell like that.

8

Lucy told me I was retarded 'cause I didn't know how to tie my shoelaces. I told her, "I'm not retarded! I'm a smart girl. Mrs. Knopf said so, go ask Mrs. Knopf." Threw my shoe at Lucy, too, but I didn't hit her. Oh, I couldn't wait to learn to read, show them kids if I was retarded or not retarded!

But Mrs. Knopf just kept learning me my alphabet and my numbers and how to write them. Over and over and over I done it. It was such hard work, all that stuff, it takes such a lot of pain being helped.

I liked to be in school; I never had no fights in school. But always I was getting in troubles in the building. Some of the kids teased me to death 'cause they knew I'm easy to get in troubles. All they have to do is say I'm not as smart as they are, call me retarded, call me a dope. Then they know I'm gonna fly at them and hit and scream, and Mrs. Drake or Mrs. Spencer is gonna have to smack me. The attendants could smack me harder than I could smack the kids. The kids liked it when I got smacked. Sometimes they laughed.

Also, I was getting in troubles from taking things. When kids got things and I didn't get things, I would have to go and take some of their stuff. Lollipops Bettyann got from her mother. I ate up three of them lollipops, all the red ones, before Bettyann seen what I was doing. Whenever the kids get goodies, I tried to take some, too. Once I even took a ring, Josephine's ring. Her mother give it to her for her birthday, or maybe it was her grandmother. It was such a pretty ring and got a teeny flower picture on it. But I couldn't wear it, couldn't let Josephine see it, so I had to keep it under my pillow and the cleaning lady found it. She give it to Mrs. Drake and Mrs. Drake come after me, yelled, "Winifred, you gotta stop taking things that isn't yours!"

"Well, what can I take?" I yell back. "Nothing is mine!"

I got a bad punishment for that. They made me set on my bed all day and didn't get my food, no lunch or supper. Just set there and be hungry all the day long. I rather be smacked.

Next day the kids was teasing me about getting punished, and while we was walking to school, Josephine kept telling everyone that Winifred is a stealer. I told her to shut up, I screamed at her, but she wouldn't stop saying Winifred is a stealer. By the time we got to school I was all upset, feeling real disturbed.

While the other kids was busy working and Mrs. Knopf was busy helping, I went outside, quiet, so no one seen me going. I knew there was poison ivy behind the school. Mrs. Knopf was always telling us about it, telling us not to go near it when we was out to play. I went right in that poison ivy, pulled off the leafs and rubbed it on my face and my arms and my legs.

When I come back Mrs. Knopf said, "Where was you, Winifred?" I told her the bathroom. She just said, "Well, next time tell me." I felt bad about lying to Mrs. Knopf. I never done that before.

At nighttime I got all over itchy, itching something awful. Miss Busby come over to my bed, said, "What's wrong with you?"

"I went in poison ivy," I said. "I went in poison ivy be-hind the school."

"Why did you do that kind of thing?"

"I don't know. Just to be smart."

My eyes got all swelled up, they had to put ice packs on my eyes. They put lotion on my face, on my legs, I was covered with lotion. They put mittens on my hands so I couldn't scratch. I wanted to scratch so bad! I had to stay in bed, and my bed was messed up with lotion all over the sheets. Couldn't go to school, just had to stay in bed cov-ered with lotion and itching so bad I couldn't keep myself still. Oh, it was terrible.

I learned my lesson. Don't touch poison ivy.

Was I glad when the day come I could go back to school, was I glad to see Mrs. Knopf again. I was still waiting to learn to read. I thought it would be such proud fun when my mother and daddy and Wanda and Miriam and Gladys seen me and I just pick up a book and start reading like anything. Was they ever gonna be surprised.

But most of the times I tried not to think about my mother and daddy and sisters no more. It made me feel too bad. Every visiting day they didn't come, and I got so sick of waiting for them that I didn't even wait no more. When it come to be visiting day I just say, "Oh, so what, visiting day. I don't care 'cause no one's gonna come." And I wouldn't wait. I'd play in the yard with Donald Duck, chasing him and quacking at him, or I'd ride the tricycle, and not pay no mind to the cars going by.

I knew they must of forgot about me, it was such a long time. And I knew my daddy wasn't gonna find where I was. I knew they didn't want me; otherwise why did they leave me here? Why didn't they come back and get me? Why didn't they even come and visit me?

Sometimes some of the girls get mail, such as a letter or postcard from their family, but I never even got that. And it would bother me, many a time it would bother me. Like, why didn't they want me, why did they forget about me? It's not nice when a family forgets about a kid, it's not fair. It makes the kid mad. It even makes the kid feel real sad and cry.

They shouldn't of done like that. They shouldn't of done like that to me.

So why should I care about them if they wasn't gonna care about me?

Jeannie's mother, when she come on visiting day, she ask Mrs. Spencer could Winifred come for a walk with her, 'cause I didn't get no company. Mrs. Spencer said yes, Winifred could go.

Jeannie's mother let me help push Jeannie up and down the driveway. I made believe she was my own mother come to visit. "Let's set on the grass," she said, so we find a nice spot and she put Jeannie down. Jeannie had to lay down, couldn't set up too good by herself. She can't help it, got poor muscles I guess.

Jeannie's mother took some cookies out of a bag in her pocketbook, give Jeannie one to chew on, she give me two. They was good cookies, with jelly in them. I gobbled them right down. But I didn't ask for more, could be she was saving them for Jeannie.

Jeannie laid there smiling. She was playing with the leafs I found for her—red leafs, yellow leafs—and chewing on her cookie. She was such a pretty little thing, big blue eyes and blonde hair all full of curls like a doll. I patted her curls. They felt good, they felt soft.

"She likes it when you sing to her," her mother told me.

"I don't know how to sing, don't know no songs to sing."

So she sing to Jeannie. Pretty songs about Jesus Christ and then some funny songs. Jeannie laughed. She couldn't understand what her mother was singing, I guess she just laughed to hear her mother's voice. I felt happy, too, listening to the pretty songs. I laid down next to Jeannie and held her little hand.

"Does your family come to see you?" Jeannie's mother ask.

"No. Nobody comes to see me."

"Then sometimes on visiting day you could walk with us."

9

One night I was laying in my bed sleeping, I was sleeping real good 'cause I got use to the noises and fits a long time ago. When you get use to them things, they hardly never bother you or wake you up. And I felt someone pulling and pulling my arm. Miss Busby. "Get up, Winifred, get up," she was saying, only real quiet. I open my eyes. It was all dark and the other kids was sleeping. Miss Busby picked me up and she carry me to Mrs. Treadwell's office. I was so sleepy I didn't know what I was doing or where I was going. Then I seen my Uncle Ned. My Uncle Ned was setting right there in Mrs. Treadwell's office.

I didn't ask what he was doing there or what they was doing with me; I still wasn't all awake. He took me and he carry me outside; he put me in a car, laid me in the back seat. It was real dark and inside the car it was cold. Uncle Ned covered me with something, like a blanket, made me warm. I just wanted to sleep. Right away I fell to sleep again.

This was so strange. Next thing I open my eyes and it was morning time, light outside, and I was home in my own bed. I thought, wait a minute. Can't be. Must be I'm having a dream about being home. I had so many of them it isn't funny. So I close my eyes again and then I open them real, real slow and peep out. Sure enough, I was still there. Wanda and Miriam was in the other beds, they was sleeping. I jump up, run to the window and looked out. I could see the big tree and the backyard and the apple trees and the garage and my mother's car. It wasn't in a dream, it was in real!

I tried to wake up Wanda and Miriam, I called them and pulled them and they set up in bed. Miriam told me, "Hi!" and Wanda right away said, "Look at her hair, look at her short hair." I was so excited. I said, "How did I get here?"

"Don't you know?"

Then I remembered about Uncle Ned, about him carrying me to the car. "Sure I know, I just forgot."

Wanda said, "How come you got your hair cut off?"

"'Cause I didn't want my braids no more," I told her. All I have to do is be with Wanda one minute, right away she says something to get me mad. I ask Miriam, "Where's Patches?"

"Patches is outside. He don't sleep in here no more."

"Where's my mother and daddy? Why did Uncle Ned come get me?"

"Daddy's in the hospital," Miriam told me. "He got another heart attack. But he's coming home today."

I run downstairs, I was still in my nightie. I could smell good kitchen smells, something yummy cooking. My mother was there, she was making cornbread, and Uncle Ned was setting at the table drinking coffee. My mother was still in her nightie, too, with her blue bathrobe and got fuzzy slippers on her feets. She seen me, said, "Well, here's Winnie."

I felt shy a little, didn't know what to say. She give me a hug. I wanted to hug her back, but I was feeling too mad at her. For leaving me there so long, for not coming to get me sooner. My mother told Uncle Ned, "See? She won't even hug me."

"When is my daddy coming home?"

"Today."

"I wanna see Patches."

"You gotta get dressed first, can't go out in your nightie. It's chilly."

Uncle Ned went and got a paper bag from the closet near the back door. Some of my clothes was in it. "Go up and get Miriam to dress you," my mother said, but I told her, "No, I could do it myself. I just gotta be buttoned." And I march upstairs and dress, then I brush my teeths myself. Was they all surprised! I felt proud I could do them things.

Out I run to find Patches. I called and called and he come running. Boy, was he glad to see me, he remembered me. He wagged his tail, he wiggle all up and down hisself, he jump on me and licked my face. Almost knocked me over. Patches is big, he's part collie, but I didn't care that he almost knocked me over. I just laughed. I was so happy to see that dog, to see Patches. We run around the backyard, we run around the garage, we run into the woods. I didn't care if I ever stopped running. I was so glad to be home, so glad to run with Patches. We went to see the chickens, and I said, "Hi, chickens, I'm home!" They just clucked. Guess they thought I come to feed them.

Then we went up on the big hill, me and Patches, where we always go. We set there on the rocks and I could see everything. Cars going by on the road, cows, our house, the apple trees, the garage, the chicken coops. I could see the whole world without the whole world seeing me. We set there until I got cold, I wasn't wearing no sweater, and I was hungry 'cause I didn't get my breakfast yet. So I said, "Come on, Patches, let's go," and we walk back through the woods. We go real slow so we could crunch the leafs. The trees was all the bright colors and the leafs on the ground was crunchy. Inside I felt happy, I felt all the bright colors in my insides, too. I felt happy to be with Patches.

★　　★　　★

We all set in the kitchen and had breakfast. I had oatmeal and cocoa and cornbread and I got seconds of cornbread. It was so good, it was still warm. I liked it that I could get seconds.

I didn't want to talk to my mother much. But she didn't pay me no heed, even Wanda didn't talk to me or tease me. Mostly they was eating and talking about my daddy. My mother and Uncle Ned was gonna go get him after breakfast. Before they left my mother told me, "When your daddy comes home, he's gotta have lots of quiet, he's gotta rest to get better. So you be good, Winnie, don't do no carrying on."

"Don't worry, I'm not gonna bother my daddy. I like my daddy, I want him to get better."

"And mind Miriam and Wanda while we're gone. Don't get in no troubles."

But I did, I did get in troubles while they was gone. From the cornbread. I was setting at the table, setting right in front of the cornbread, and I thought, hmmmm, maybe I could take a little more. Miriam turned around, she and Wanda was doing the dishes, and she seen my mouth full. She got mad at me, told me, "Leave that cornbread alone, Winnie. You already had plenty!" I couldn't say nothing, I put too much in my mouth.

"Look how much she took," Wanda said. "She wasn't gonna leave none for daddy. She shouldn't even be here, she's just gonna bother him to death."

"I am not gonna bother him to death!" I hollered when I got my mouth working.

"Well, you're starting up already. That's why mommy didn't want you to come home. But she had to let you come 'cause daddy wanted to see you!"

"Shut up, Wanda," Miriam said, but I was already out the door, didn't hear no more. I was running, Patches was behind me. I just wanted to get away from them. Wanda was so mean to me. It wasn't fair that she was pretty. I know that's why my mother liked Wanda best, 'cause she was pretty, I know that's why my mother bought Wanda nice clothes but not nice clothes for me. And she wasn't even Wanda's real mother, neither.

Patches and me set up on that hill a long time. The wind started up to blowing and I was getting cold, but we set there until I seen my mother's car come into the backyard. I could see my mother and Uncle Ned get out; they was helping my daddy. He was walking real slow.

When I got to the house I yelled, "Daddy! Daddy! Daddy!" and I run to him. I forgot he was sick, forgot I had to be careful. My mother said, "Winnie, don't hug him so hard."

"That's okay, Winnie could hug me," my daddy said, "'cause I didn't see her in such a long time. Look how big Winnie growed." Hugged me back, too. Then he had to go lay down. He laid down on the sofa in the living room, and I set with him while my mother made lunch. He told me, "Oh, Winnie, your hair looks nice."

"I could write some of my letters now, daddy, wanna see?" I got a pencil and paper from my mother and I set there with him drawing some letters. He said that was real good, what I was doing.

Miriam brung him his lunch on a tray—he ate on the sofa—but I had to eat in the kitchen with everybody else. Then my daddy took a nap on the sofa. My mother made him a special bed there so he could sleep downstairs, so he didn't have to go up the stairs, to help his heart get better. That's how she done before when he got his other heart attack, he slept in the living room a long time.

Gladys come to see me while my daddy was sleeping. She was near to grown up, she lived in town and she worked at the grocery store. Gladys was my favorite sister and I was Gladys's favorite sister. She had red hair, bright red hair. I always wished I could have red hair like she got, but mine is brown.

She had a bag with her. She open it up, took out a box of

gingersnaps, said, "See, I didn't forget." Always when she come she brung me gingersnaps from her store, she knows I really do love gingersnaps. I said, "Thank you!" and right away I start gobbling them up.

"I like how your hair looks," she told me. "It's more easy if you got short hair instead of long hair. Not so much brushing."

I showed her my letters I could write, like A, B, C, and D, and she come in the bathroom with me to see how good I could brush my teeths now. She praised me, said, "Oh, Winnie, that's good. You learned so much."

When my daddy got awake she wanted to see him for a little while, then she had to go. Told me, "You be a good girl, Winnie."

I said, "I will, I'll be a good girl." But I wasn't too sure about that, I always had lots of troubles trying to be a good girl. Sometimes it didn't work out.

After supper I set with my daddy for awhile—we was all listening to some radio programs—then my mother told Miriam to take me upstairs and put me to bed.

"Could Patches sleep on my bed tonight?"

"No, he's use to being outside now. We don't want him to get use to being inside again."

I didn't think that was fair, that Patches had to stay outside. It was cold, too. I stomp upstairs with Miriam.

I laid in my bed a long time waiting for Wanda and Miriam to come up. It was such a comfy bed, it felt so good to me. And quiet. No noises and fits, no kids screaming. I could hear the radio downstairs, I could hear my mother and daddy and Uncle Ned talking a little, I could hear the wind. I didn't want to go to sleep, just wanted to lay there in my bed in my room, listen to all them quiet things. When Wanda and Miriam come up they said, "You better get to sleep, you got another long trip tomorrow."

"What long trip?"

"Uncle Ned's gotta take you back tomorrow," Miriam said.

"I'm going back? I'm not going back there." I thought maybe Miriam was teasing me.

"Yes, you are," Wanda said. She told Miriam, "Winnie thinks she's staying here. Nobody told Winnie she wasn't staying here."

"I am too staying. I'm not going back there, nobody's taking me back there!"

Wanda was putting on her nightie, she just smiled at me nasty. I jumped out of bed and kicked her, kicked her right in the stomach, told her, "You're lying!" She pushed me in the face, made me fall back on my bed. I could hear my mother running upstairs.

"What's all this racket, what are you kids doing?"

"She kicked me!" Wanda said.

"Winnie, you're gonna get such a spanking if you start carrying on here," my mother told me.

"They said I was going back tomorrow!"

My mother yelled at Miriam and Wanda then, said why did they tell me that tonight, didn't they know I was gonna make troubles? They shut up, didn't say nothing to her.

"Now you get in bed too, Winnie, and no more yelling, no more kicking. Or it's gonna bother your daddy and he'll get sick again."

So I got in my bed and I was very quiet, quiet as I could be. I didn't want my daddy to get sick again. And Wanda and Miriam was quiet, too.

Before breakfast my mother put my stuff back in the paper bag, my nightie and my toothbrush and the extra dress and bloomers I got. I put in the box of gingersnaps Gladys give me, what was left. I didn't say nothing, didn't want to talk to nobody when I ate my breakfast. Wanda and Miriam had to go to the school bus.

My mother said, "Do you wanna say good-bye to your sisters?"

I said, "No."

Uncle Ned went to the garage to start the car. Sometimes it took a long time to get that car started. My mother went upstairs and come back with a green sweater of Wanda's that didn't fit her no more. She told me to put it on 'cause I didn't have no sweater or jacket with me. She buttoned me.

"Go say good-bye to your daddy," she said.

I said, "No."

"Winnie, Winnie, why do you gotta act like this?"

But I wouldn't talk to her, just stood there in the kitchen with my bag, waiting for Uncle Ned. Didn't say good-bye to her, just went out with Uncle Ned and got into the car.

I seen Patches, he was standing in the driveway wagging his tail. But I didn't even say good-bye to Patches.

10

I set in school and I didn't want to do my work. Didn't want to do nothing.

"Winifred, practice your letters," Mrs. Knopf told me. But I just set there gloomy as an old dog, didn't even pick up my pencil. Mrs. Knopf come back to me, said, "Something's wrong. What happened, Winifred? Didn't you have a good time at home?" And then I put my head down on my desk and cried.

"Winifred's crying," Edith told the other kids real loud.

Mrs. Knopf, she didn't even get mad at me, she was so nice. Just said, "Come with me, Winifred." She told the other kids to keep doing their work, she put Shirley in charge, took me to another room where there wasn't no one in it. She set with me.

"Are you sad 'cause you miss your family, Winifred? Your mother and daddy?"

"Why should I care? They don't care about me. They don't even let me stay home, they sent me away again!"

"Don't you know why you're here?"

"'Cause they don't want me in the house. Maybe they think I'm retarded or something." Mrs. Knopf had to give me her hanky, my nose was running so bad.

"You're here 'cause you need special help," she said. "Special help to learn things. You're learning so much already 'cause you're a smart girl. You could dress yourself, you could even write some of your letters. You couldn't do them things before you come here."

"But I can't read!"

"Well, that takes a long time, but you're gonna learn to read, too, Winifred. Just got to work a lot."

"Even *Cinderella*? Could I learn to read books like *Cinderella* and the one about the gingersnap boy?" Those was my favorite stories that Gladys read to me, they had them books in her store and she give them to me for my birthday once. Or Christmas. I thought Cinderella was beautiful. I wanted to be like Cinderella.

"Sure, Winifred, sure you could read them books. Just give it time."

So maybe my mother didn't like me. So what? Mrs. Knopf liked me. That made me feel better. Also made me work real hard. I was learning my letters good, could almost write my alphabet. I was learning my numbers, too.

Then Mrs. Knopf showed me how to write my name. I worked and worked, but it was hard to do. So many letters. I had to remember which letters go into my name and which letters don't go into my name. And writing the "W" was hard. It didn't always turn out the right way.

I took a paper and pencil back to the building and while the other kids was playing in the yard, I set on the ground, practiced and practiced. So I could write my name. So I could go to school and show Mrs. Knopf I could write my name. The other kids, they all said, "Look at Winifred setting there writing, she thinks she's so smart." But I didn't care. All I cared about was writing my name.

And the next day I went back to school and said, "Look, Mrs. Knopf!" I set down at my desk, picked my pencil right up, wrote "WINIFRED." Didn't even do the "W" wrong, got the whole thing right.

Mrs. Knopf said, "You done good, Winifred. I'm proud of you."

Oh, I felt so big, I felt so smart, I felt like I wasn't even retarded at all!

AUTUMN
1942

11

A new girl come while we was eating lunch. Mrs. Drake brung her down to the dining room.

"Set next to Winifred," she told her. "Winifred, this here's Antonia."

Antonia set down next to me. She didn't look too happy. She was a big girl, bigger than me. Mostly, new girls is little girls. Mrs. Drake went to get Antonia some lunch from the kitchen ladies, put it down in front of her, went back upstairs. Antonia just set there.

I said, "Aren't you gonna eat your lunch?"

Antonia didn't say nothing. I ate all my lunch, it was good. Cheese sandwich. I love cheese sandwiches.

I ask Antonia, "Could I eat your lunch?" Still she didn't say nothing, so must be she didn't mind. After I ate Antonia's sandwich, I drunk up all her milk. You could tell she didn't want her milk, neither. Mrs. Drake, when she come back, she told Antonia she was glad she ate her lunch. I wasn't gonna tell that I ate it, might get Antonia in troubles.

Mrs. Drake took Antonia back upstairs, and when she come out to the yard her hair was cut off. That's how they always do to new girls. Too many kids in Children's Cottage, it's more easier for the attendants if the kids got short hair. They don't have time to do all that brushing and braiding, they got enough work.

Antonia looked strange with her hair cut off. She had real curly hair, now it looked like fuzz on her head. Fuzzy stuff. I told her, "You look strange with hair like fuzzy stuff." Antonia just laid down on the grass.

"Why you laying on the grass, new girl?" Helen ask her.

Antonia started to cry, said, "I wanna go home!"

"You can't go home," Estelle Sampson told her. "You can't go home 'cause you're retarded."

Antonia throwed up, throwed up all over the grass. Then she throwed up again. It's a good thing she didn't eat her lunch. It would of made her even sicker.

12

"Can I go over to Forest for a little while to visit Jeannie?" I ask Mrs. Drake. You could see Jeannie's yard from our yard, and on nice days I could see Jeannie setting out there. I always try to ask Mrs. Drake, not Mrs. Spencer, and mostly Mrs. Drake tells me yes, yes you could go. I went to see Jeannie whenever I got the chance. I promised her mother I would look out for her, help take care of her. I know that made her mother real happy, that I would help take care of her.

Jeannie couldn't walk or talk. She was real retarded, even had to wear diapers like the real retarded ones did. But she looked so pretty, blonde hair and blue eyes like her mother got. She didn't look retarded.

So off I go to Forest. The other low-grades was out there, too, most of them in wheeling chairs and some was laying on the grass or on mats. Lots of them was grown up, but they act like babies, little born babies, got to have diapers, got to have bibs for the slobbering. Like Jeannie. But they wasn't pretty like Jeannie, Jeannie was the only one that was pretty. Some look so awful you don't even want to see them, you get a sick feeling inside. I tried not to look at the others too much, only wanted to look at Jeannie.

I said, "Hi, Jeannie!" She smiled when she seen me and made happy little baby noises. I ask the attendant if I could lift her out of the wheeling chair. I was trying to learn her to walk.

"You could pick her up," the attendant said, "but she's not gonna do no walking." That's what the attendant always said.

So I pick up Jeannie real gentle, lift her out of her wheeling chair, and I hold her under her arms and try to get her to move her little feets. She give me a look, then she laughed. I loved the way her laugh sounded, it always made me feel good to hear her laughing. She said, "Mama!" She could say "mama." But she didn't move her feets, she thought it was a game we was playing.

The attendant laughed too, said, "When are you gonna give it up, Winifred?"

I told her, "Well, maybe she can't walk, and maybe she is retarded, but I still like her."

When I left I waved bye-bye at Jeannie and she waved bye-bye at me. Jeannie knew how to wave bye-bye, her mother learned her. She looked so cute when she done that. She knew it, too.

One of them low-grades—a big fat one in a wheeling chair—she seen me waving so she had to wave, too. She didn't hardly have no hair and got no teeths almost, but there she was, setting in her wheeling chair waving at me, setting there in her big diapers and shirt looking happy as an old goose.

I wished she wouldn't do like that, wave at me and go, "Bye, bye, bye, bye, bye."

13

It rained and rained a long time, days and days of raining out. We couldn't go outside, only to school, had to stay in the building in the playroom every day after school. I hate that, all them noises from the kids gets on my nerves. I got bad nerves. And it don't always smell too good when everyone is inside.

I try to keep myself busy, look at books, do puzzles, crayon pictures, I try to pay no heed to the others. When everyone is inside the kids carry on more, they tease you worse. Sometimes the kids made fun of me 'cause I couldn't talk clear. Even kids that don't talk good make fun of other kids that don't talk good. Call them dumb or retarded, say they talk baby talk. And that bothered me, that really did bother me. 'Cause most of all I didn't want to be mentally retarded.

I told Antonia, "I'm gonna fix it so no one would think I'm mentally retarded." Antonia was a good kid to talk to. She just listened, she didn't talk much. But when she did, she talked real good. I told her, "I wish I could talk like you. You talk so clear that people could understand you."

She said, "Why don't you get help?"

"Who to?"

But Antonia didn't say nothing after that, just set there putting beads on her string. Lots of times she wouldn't answer you. I guess she couldn't think of enough things to say.

Hmmmmm, I thought, maybe Mrs. Knopf could help me. She could help with anything. So when I went to school, I ask her, "Mrs. Knopf, could you help me with my speech? I want to talk like people who could talk clear, so the kids won't call me retarded."

Mrs. Knopf said yes, yes she could help me, and while

the kids was having playtime, she start off making sounds like "B" and "T" and she tell me to do like she do. I tried but it was too hard. My mouth didn't work good enough.

"You just keep practicing them sounds, Winifred," she told me. "Then I'll do more sounds for you to practice."

After school I set in the playroom and practiced. Tried to make them sounds with my mouth like Mrs. Knopf showed me. Right away the kids started dogging me, teasing and laughing.

"Don't bother me," I told them. "I'm learning to talk clear." But they kept going at me. Didn't have nothing better to do on rainy days. And Estelle Sampson copied me, copied every sound I was trying to make. That got me mad. She could make them sounds without even practicing.

"Stop it!" I told her, but she wouldn't stop it. "Shut up!" I told her, but she wouldn't shut up. I picked up a puzzle and threw it at her. All the pieces come flying out every which way and the board, the wooden board, hit her in the head. She come after me yowling like something wild, she grab me and start banging me up against the wall. Bang, bang, bang, she goes with me. It wasn't fair, I couldn't fight back. I was little and skinny and she was big and fat.

By the time the attendants come my nose was bleeding, also had a cut lip and a bumped-up arm. It took two attendants and Mrs. Treadwell to pull Estelle Sampson away from me, and she was still yowling and kicking. They had to put her in a straitjacket, tie her up good and tight. Straitjackets are for girls who get really disturbed. Straitjackets keep them still until they can be calm down, act polite again, straitjackets keep them from hurting other people and theirselfs.

While they was tying up Estelle Sampson, the cleaning lady give me a wet cloth for my nose, stop the bleeding. I was shaking, I was crying something hysterical. They had to give me medicine and put me to bed. I was a mess, my nerves was all scrambled up. After I was in bed, after I was quiet, Mrs. Treadwell come to see if I was feeling better.

She told me, "I gotta give you a punishment for throwing that puzzle, Winifred, for hitting Estelle Sampson. And your punishment is for you to stay in the building one week. You can't go out, can't even go to school. Just stay in and think what you done."

I said, "Okay, Mrs. Treadwell. Could I have some juice now?" So she told Mrs. Spencer to get Winifred some juice, I was real thirsty. I think the medicine they give you does that, or maybe it comes from getting too disturbed.

Estelle Sampson didn't have to stay in. They took her someplace. She was away for awhile, but I don't know where. I hate Estelle Sampson. I hate her big head.

Mrs. Spencer kept me in a long time. Much longer than a week. She wasn't suppose to do like that, but she didn't care. She done lots of things she wasn't suppose to do. Once she even pushed a kid, pushed Angela, and that made her fall down the stairs. Mrs. Spencer told Mrs. Treadwell that Angela tripped. But me and Helen seen it. Angela wasn't smart enough to tell what happened, she was one of the real dopey kids, and we wasn't gonna tell neither. We knew Mrs. Spencer would come after us. She would kill us.

I ask Mrs. Drake, "When could I go outside again? When could I go to school? 'Cause it's a long time already and I'm still in the building."

She said, "I don't know, Winifred." But while the other kids was in school, I was in the playroom and I heard them talking about it in the dining room when they was having their coffee. Mrs. Spencer told Mrs. Drake to keep out of it; Mrs. Spencer told Mrs. Drake, "I'm taking care of it."

And it wasn't raining no more, neither. It was all nice and sunshiny out and I was sick of being in that darn building. I needed to go outside, I needed fresh air. I heard a kid could get sick if she didn't get her fresh air.

I went to Mrs. Spencer. I told her, "Mrs. Spencer, when could I go out?"

"When I say so, that's when."

"But I need my fresh air or I'm gonna come down sick."

"No, you won't."

So I had to start sneaking. When the kitchen ladies was gone, I could go out the kitchen door, up the steps, then I was outside. I stand there and sniff the air, smile at the sky, feel that sunshine on me; then I sneak back down the stairs. No one ever seen me coming or going. And that's how I got my fresh air.

One morning I was doing it—the other kids was in school and I was standing outside by the kitchen steps—and I heard music. Lots of music, loud music. I thought, oh, I gotta find that music! I forgot all about I was sneaking out, forgot about what would happen if they catched me, just took off after that music. It sounded like it was calling to me, it was so joyful.

A bunch of grown-up girls was standing on the front lawn looking over the big hedge. The music was coming from the other side, the music was coming from the road. And they was all in a dither, clapping and waving, and one girl was dancing. I tried to look over, too, but I couldn't, I was too little. Even when I stood on tippytoes, my eyes couldn't reach. So I crawl into the hedge—there was a hole. I set in there and peeped out from the leafs and I seen a parade, a parade going by on the road. People and soldier men and even some kids in the most beautiful sparkly clothes, they was all marching along together to that music. They got flags and shiny horns and big drums. I wondered where did that kind of people come from, where did that kind of people live? I don't remember if I knew what it was then, don't remember if I knew it was a parade. I think I just thought it was some kind of magic.

When they was all gone down the road to town, when everything was quiet and plain again, I run back to Children's Cottage. I wanted to tell somebody so bad, wanted to tell Ruby Rose or Antonia what a wonderful thing I seen. But I didn't. I knew they was gonna say I was lying.

*　　*　　*

I got a letter from my daddy. I was so thrilled. He wrote me a couple times, and I saved his letters. Also Gladys sent me a birthday card once. I kept all my letters in my Belongings Box, I think I had four letters by then. Some kids had one letter, some kids had two letters, some kids didn't have none. But I must of had around four.

I had to get someone to read the letter for me, I couldn't read. Reading is very hard, reading takes a long time to learn. So I asked Shirley to read it to me. She was one of the big kids, she was the best reader. She could read my daddy's letter to me real good. My daddy said he was fine and my mother was fine, and Wanda and Miriam and Gladys was all fine.

"So what," I said, "so what if Wanda's fine?" Shirley kept reading. He said the chickens was fine. He said he missed me and he hoped I was being a good girl at the institution. It was a fine letter. I put it right in my Belongings Box.

More days passed, then more and more days, and still I was staying inside the building. Not going to school, not going out to play. Had to set around by myself and mess with the puzzles, do beads, blocks, look out the window.

I told Miss Kolski—she's the attendant who comes when Mrs. Drake has her days off—I told Miss Kolski I didn't have nothing to do. Kept complaining all morning, so she give me a broom and told me to sweep out the dorm, said, "That'll give you something to do."

"I don't wanna sweep. I wanna go outside."

Mrs. Spencer come over, told me, "You do what Miss Kolski says."

But I wouldn't, I wouldn't sweep. Miss Kolski tried to put the broom in my hand and I wouldn't take it. It fell on the floor. She said, "Pick it up," but I didn't move. Mrs. Spencer tried to smack me, but I duck down real quick so I wouldn't get hit, cussed her out, too. I was learning lots of bad words from the big kids.

Mrs. Spencer flyed into a fury when I cussed her, said,

"Okay, Winifred, you act like an animal so I'm gonna treat you like an animal!" and she took me by the arm and pulled me downstairs to the dining room. I had to go with her, I didn't have no choice. She told one of the kitchen ladies, "Give me some lunch for Winifred!"

The lady took a plate and put some spaghetti on it, put a meatball on top of the spaghetti, give it to Mrs. Spencer. Mrs. Spencer put the plate on the floor in the corner and told me, "Now eat your food like an animal." She tried to push me down on the floor by the plate, but I wouldn't go down. I was frightened, but I wasn't gonna set on the floor and eat my spaghetti with just my mouth, without no spoon.

"I'm not gonna do that!" I told her. "I don't have to do that!"

"Well, you're gonna set there till you do."

"I'll get back at you," I hollered. "I'll tell everything I know!" She just stomp upstairs to get the other kids for lunch. Boy, I could of ratted on her, could of got her in so much trouble. But I guess she knew I'd never do it.

When Mrs. Spencer come back with the other kids, she seen me still standing there. She come over like to hit me, so I set down real quick by the plate. But I didn't eat. Some of the kids looked at me, they knew what was going on. They seen Mrs. Spencer do that to other kids when she got real mad. But they didn't say nothing, just ate their lunch. Nobody wanted to get Mrs. Spencer mad at them.

I set there and looked at my spaghetti until lunchtime was over. It smelled so good, that meatball looked so good. And my stomach was all growly, making noises like anything. I love spaghetti. But I wasn't gonna eat it. I heard a saying: you could lead an animal to water but you can't make him eat it. Mrs. Spencer could make me set there, but she couldn't make me eat like an animal.

After all the kids was gone to the yard and the tables was cleaned and the kitchen ladies left, I snuck into the pantry. Way up high on the tippytop shelf was a big box of graham crackers. Oh boy, was I hungry. I ask myself, hmmmm, can I get up that far or can't I get up that far? The answer come back yes, yes I can get up that far.

I put one foot on one shelf and another foot on another shelf. Oops, knocked over a big can. It went bang on the floor. I wait real still with my feets on the shelf, but no one come. Wasn't no one down there to hear it, I guess.

Then I reached up way high to grab the graham cracker box and, darn it, I knocked that graham cracker box down, too. But it didn't go bang like the can. I set on the pantry floor and ate a whole bunch of crackers. Then I put some in my dress pocket 'cause maybe I was gonna get hungry again later.

While Miss Kolski was washing my head and I was bended over the sink, she seen the graham crackers in my pocket. She said, "What's that in your pocket?"

"Graham crackers."

"Where did you get them?"

"I took them. From the pantry."

She finished washing, got all the soap out, rubbed my head with a towel to get it dry. She told the next kid in line to wait and she brung me to Mrs. Treadwell's office. She took some of the crackers out of my pocket and showed Mrs. Treadwell, said, "Look what I found in Winifred's pocket."

"What are you doing with them crackers, Winifred?" Mrs. Treadwell ask me.

"I'm gonna eat them."

"Who give them to you?"

"Nobody give them to me. I took them. I was hungry."

"Didn't you eat? Didn't you get your lunch?"

So I told her what happened, told her Mrs. Spencer wanted me to eat off the floor like an animal, but I wouldn't do it. Mrs. Treadwell told Miss Kolski to go get Mrs. Spencer. And when she come in Mrs. Treadwell ask her, "Why did you try to make Winifred eat off the floor?"

"Well, she carries on all the time."

I said, "You'd carry on too if you wanted to go out for fresh air!"

"Why can't you go out for fresh air?" Mrs. Treadwell said.

"Don't ask me," I told her. "You're the one punished me."

"That was last month, Winifred. I said you gotta stay in the building one week."

"Well, I been in the building since then, not even out to school."

Mrs. Treadwell give Mrs. Spencer such a look. I could tell Mrs. Spencer was in trouble. Mrs. Treadwell told me, "Okay, Winifred, go down and get your supper now."

I went out of the room. When I pass Mrs. Spencer, I give her a big smile. I knew she wasn't gonna be bothering me for awhile. She wasn't gonna dare.

I closed the door, the office door, stood out there listening. I heard Mrs. Treadwell say, "She's only a little kid, ten years old. She needs to go outside, she needs to go to school. You got no rights to be keeping her in the building!"

Then I heard someone coming, so I run down to get my supper.

And I still got three crackers left in my pocket.

14

First thing when I went back to school I told Mrs. Knopf, "I got a letter from my daddy. Could you help me write to him? 'Cause I never done a letter before."

I had a lot of work, a whole lot of work to do to get catched up from missing so much school, but when playtime come Mrs. Knopf let me stay inside and she helped me make a letter for my daddy. I could write all my alphabet, but I couldn't spell much, only little words I could spell such as "cat" and "go." I didn't need to put "cat" or "go" into my letter, so Mrs. Knopf had to spell everything for me. I told her what I wanted to say, she told me how to spell it. And I print so careful with my pencil, I done neat as I could. I told my daddy I was fine, I told my daddy I missed him. I told my daddy I got a friend name Jeannie I take care of. I told my daddy to please come visit me soon as he could.

They did come once, my mother and daddy come to see me once. But it was a long time ago, and they didn't even take me nowhere. Just set with me on the grass awhile. Talked to me. My daddy told me Patches died. He was sick, Patches was, then Miriam went in the garage and seen him in there dead. When I heard that, I cried. I bet Patches never would of died if they hadn't sent me away. If I was home, I would of taken care of Patches; if I was home, he'd still be sleeping on my bed all alive and warm.

After they told me about Patches, they told me more things about home, like what everyone was doing, and they ask me things, like what was I doing. I ask them things, too, like when could I come home? My mother said, "Some day."

"Which day is some day?

"I don't know yet," she said. "Let's take a walk."

So we go for a walk and I showed them my school where I was gonna learn to read, and they buyed me a soda at the canteen. Then they said they better be leaving 'cause they got a long way to go to get home.

Didn't bring me nothing, no goodies or toys. Just sad news about Patches. But I still wanted them to come back. Take me to a restaurant like some of the other kids do with their families. I never been in a restaurant. And I wanted them to bring me a toy, such as a doll, or some candy for me to eat. I wanted to get company so bad. No one ever come to visit me but that one time.

Mrs. Knopf went to the office to get my daddy's address. I didn't know the address, didn't even know what town. And she wrote all that on the envelope and I licked the stamp. Did that envelope ever look important! My daddy was gonna be so proud; could be he'd come right away to see me.

I said, "Mrs. Knopf, do you think when my daddy gets that letter and reads about that I want him to come visit me, do you think he'll come?" I thought maybe that's how you get company. By letters.

"I don't know, Winifred," she said. "No way of telling."

Next visiting day there I was, setting out in the yard waiting. I sent a letter to my daddy and he read it, he read what I said to him, that I want him to come. So maybe he was really gonna come.

I set in that darn yard all day and waited. Lucy's family come and Antonia's family come and Ruby Rose's mother come. No one else. My daddy didn't come.

Mrs. Knopf said maybe he didn't get my letter yet.

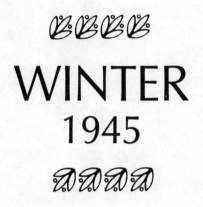

WINTER
1945

15

It was snowing hard, a real snowstorm. We was in the playroom, we was standing on chairs looking out the high windows at all the snow coming down to the ground.

"Oh, can't we go out, can't we go out?" Gloria kept asking. She was one of the little kids, one of the newer kids.

"No, you can't go out," Mrs. Drake told her.

"I wanna play in the snow," Gloria said. But we wasn't allowed to play in the snow. I know why, 'cause there wasn't enough snow clothes for all of us. We could go to school, put boots on, but we wasn't allowed to get all full of snow, get all wet and cold.

We sure was tired of being inside. You spend a lot of time in the playroom in winter, can't use the yard so much. You get tired of coloring and doing puzzles if you gotta do that all the time. Anyway, I was sick of the puzzles. I done them all long ago and we never got new ones. Same old dumb puzzles.

Some days a lady come to play records for us. That was fun. And sometimes another lady come to help us make scrapbooks. I cut out pictures of pretty ladies from the magazines she gives us, pretty ladies with pretty clothes, to paste in my scrapbook. Also, sometimes Mrs. Knopf lets me take a book home from school and I try to read. I could read some of the words if it's a real easy book.

Ruby Rose yelled, "Look, look out the window," and we seen two men coming up the walk, they was pulling a big tree.

Then we knew Christmas was coming!

We heard bump, bump, bump, and swish, swish, swish, and that was the tree coming down the stairs. It was all covered with snow, so was the men, and snow was falling off making little puddles all over the playroom floor. That tree smelled so good, smelled so darn good, we all sniff and sniff it. Smelled to me like woods and outside and running.

After it was stood up in the stand, we shout, "Can we decorate? Can we decorate now?" Oh, we was excited. Mrs. Spencer give us paper, red and green paper, and scissors for the bigger kids like me. I'm real good at chains. We cut the paper in long pieces, first the red and then the green, and the littler kids get to help glue it together to make the chains real long. When we got the chains put together, we hang them all over the tree, have to stand on chairs to do it. We also make other decorations with paper and glue and yarn, such as birds and snowmans. Ruby Rose made a big star out of yellow paper. Josephine, she's the tallest girl, she stood on a chair and stuck it on top of the tree.

What a beautiful Christmas tree!

"Could I go downstairs a minute? Could I see the tree again before I go to sleep?"

Mrs. O'Brien, she was one of the night attendants, she was a little bit mean and a little bit nice, she said, "Okay, hurry up."

Down I run and there was the tree, and I just stood there so I could look and look, and smell the outdoor smell. That whole room smelled of the outdoor smell. It put me in mind of when I was little, when I lived with my mother and daddy. Daddy would get me all dressed up warm, even to a cap on my head and a scarf on my neck, and off we would go through the woods with Patches to pick out our Christmas tree.

When we find just the right one, my daddy would tell me, "Stand back, Winnie, stand way back," and chop, chop he would go with his axe. Like when he cut off the chickens' heads, only trees take a whole lot more chopping than chickens do. And he'd chop for a long time and down would come that tree. Daddy would carry it home while Patches and me run behind, Patches barking something joyful like he knew Christmas was coming.

Then I thought, no more Patches. Patches went into the garage and he died.

I got to feeling funny all over and I run back upstairs real quick and got into my bed.

16

Mrs. Knopf let us sing Christmas carols. Some of the kids didn't know them, some of the kids did know them. I did, I knew all my carols. I love to sing them. I love "Oh, Little Town of Bethlehem" and "Away in a Manger," but my very best carol is "Silent Night." It's so beautiful, it's touchable.

After school I ask for special permission to go over to Forest, see Jeannie, see if she's got a Christmas tree yet. I didn't see Jeannie for awhile, it was so cold and snowy everyone been inside a long time. So I wait for Mrs. Drake to come downstairs—I wasn't gonna ask Mrs. Spencer—and Mrs. Drake said I could go.

I put on my boots, I put on my coat, out I go in all that snow. I love to walk in the snow, your feets goes down deep and makes a shush-shush sound.

When I got to Forest, right away I smelled that smell. It's awful in Forest Building, smells like toilets. And it's so noisy it makes our building seem quiet, you could hear all them low-grades screaming and crying and fussing. I wouldn't even go in there ever if I didn't want to see Jeannie so bad.

"Hello, Winifred," the attendants say. They all know me 'cause I'm such a friend of Jeannie's.

"I want to see Jeannie, where's Jeannie?"

"She's not here. She's in the hospital."

I got scared. "What happened?"

"She had to go get all her teeths pulled out."

"Why did she have to do that?"

"On account of her gums wasn't healthy. They made her teeths go bad."

Poor Jeannie. What a terrible thing.

When Jeannie got out of the hospital next day, they let me go see her. Her mother, Mrs. McKenna, was there. I liked Mrs. McKenna and she liked me; I guess she liked the way I always tried to help with Jeannie. You could say Mrs. McKenna was my friend and I was Mrs. McKenna's friend.

"Hi, Winifred," she said. She was setting in a chair by Jeannie's crib. They got big cribs in Forest 'cause most of the low-grades are grown up. They got big cribs, big diapers, even big playpens. Mrs. McKenna was knitting, knitting something purple. She looked real tired, like she wasn't getting her rest, but she still looked pretty. "What are you doing here?" she ask me.

"I come to see Jeannie. I heard she was in the hospital."

Jeannie was laying in her crib, crying and crying. She looked strange with all her teeths gone, she looked different. Sometimes Mrs. McKenna would put her knitting down, stand up and pat Jeannie, talk to her real soft, try to get her to stop all her crying and fretting. But it didn't work. I tried to make Jeannie stop crying, too. I wave at her through the bars and I tickle her tummy. But nothing would stop that crying.

I felt bad, felt real bad for Jeannie. She was such a pretty little thing and now she looked awful funny with all her teeths gone.

⋆　　⋆　　⋆

Christmas Eve we march over to the Assembly Hall for Christmas services. We was feeling so gay. We sang carols while an old lady played the piano, we said prayers and heard about Jesus Christ and how he got born in a stable. When I was real little, I didn't have no faith, didn't know what God was. Then I seen pictures of the Lord, they showed movies in the Assembly Hall with pictures of the Lord. He had white hair and a long beard. I said, "Is that what God looks like?" They said, "Yes, that's what God looks like." And there was pictures of what the Lord does, and a lady was singing, and oh, it was so beautiful. So I ask the lady from the church, "Is there really a God?"

"Sure there is," she told me.

"Will He help me?"

"Yes. Just give Him a chance."

I told her, "Okay. I'm gonna start believing in things." And the next time Estelle Sampson smacked me I said, "You're gonna get your day for hitting me, you just wait. God is good. He's slow but He's sure. He'll get you."

Best of all I like the Virgin Mother. She watches over people, she answers prayers. But I know it takes a lot of time for your prayers to be answered.

Now I go to church every Sunday in the Assembly Hall, also go on special holidays like Easter and Christmas.

When we come back to the building it was late, time for bed, and all the kids was talking, buzzing and buzzing, about what kind of present they was gonna get Christmas morning. Some of the kids thought Santa Claus was coming to the institution, but the rest of us know where the presents really come from. Mr. Buckholz, he's superintendent of the whole institution, he gets the money and he sends people out to buy presents for all the kids and grownup girls. Except for the low-grades. 'Cause they don't know the difference.

We all brush our teeths and get into our nighties, the

smarter girls and the attendants help the ones that can't dress theirselfs. And we all get into bed. But I couldn't fall to sleep. It wasn't the noises, I was use to the girls crying and yelling in their sleep. Sometimes they tell me I yell and cry in my sleep, too. I was feeling sad, that's why I couldn't sleep. I love Christmastime, but sometimes it makes me feel so sad inside, it makes me think of Christmastime at home. When I was little, I use to believe in Santa Claus. I peeked, I peeked on the stairs, I can remember that. Wanted to see if there was a real Santa or if there wasn't a real Santa. It was my daddy. I seen him putting some presents under the tree. When he turn around, I run upstairs fast as a little chickie. He thought I was still sleeping.

They give me dominos for Christmas once and Gladys tried to show me how to do the dominos, but I just couldn't get the hang of it. Couldn't count all them darn spots, they always got me mixed up. So I used them to build. I builded a little house with them; I builded a chicken coop with them. Or I would stand them up in a row, then knock them over and laugh to see them all fall down.

Also got hair ribbons for Christmas one time. I think Gladys or Miriam give them to me. They was red and green and Gladys tied them in my braids Christmas morning and I felt pretty as a Christmas tree, all red and green. My mother and daddy had a tree with lights, real lights that lit up. That was the most beautiful thing. We didn't have no lights on our tree at the institution, only just chains and decorations such as we make of paper.

I laid in bed and always in my thoughts was home, my Christmastime at home, and all of the sudden I bust out in tears. I wanted to go home so bad. Some of the kids, their families took them home for Christmas. Nobody ever took me home. I didn't even hear from no one, didn't get no mail for such a long time, seemed like everyone forgot me. I wanted them to remember me. I wanted to be home. I didn't want to be in the institution.

★   ★   ★

My Christmas present was a game of cards. It was called "Go Fishing." I was setting there trying to figure out how you work it when Mrs. Spencer come to me, said, "Winifred, Mrs. Treadwell wants to see you. Go to her office."

I thought, uh-oh, what did I do now? But I couldn't think of nothing bad I done, nothing so bad to get sent to Mrs. Treadwell.

Mrs. Treadwell told me, "Set down, Winifred," so I set down. Then she told me, "Yesterday Mrs. McKenna called me. She's coming tomorrow to get Jeannie, take her home for a visit. She wants to know if you want to go, too."

"Go home with Mrs. McKenna to visit?"

"Yes."

"For a long time? And sleep at her house?"

"For a couple days."

"Oh boy, oh boy!" What a thrill!

In the afternoon we went to the Assembly Hall again, hear some of the grown-up girls singing Christmas songs. Then a man, a man who was dressed up like Santa Claus, he give everybody goodies to eat. Cookies and candy. And we all sing "Jingle Bells." It was real fun, I had a good time, but mostly I was just waiting to hurry up and get to tomorrow.

In the morning Mrs. Spencer put some of my stuff in a bag. Clothes, toothbrush, hairbrush, things like that. And I put in my new cards. I thought maybe Mrs. McKenna might show me how to work it, play that game, when we got to her house. Mrs. Davis took me over to Forest to meet Mrs. McKenna, she had her car out front and one of the attendants was helping her get Jeannie in the back seat. She said, "Merry Christmas, Winifred! Are you all ready to go?"

"I sure am!" I told her.

Mrs. McKenna looked so pretty, like always, and her fur coat looked so soft I wanted to touch it, wanted the feel of it.

"You could set in front, Winifred."

"Oh, goody."

I waved bye-bye to Mrs. Davis, then off we go. It was a nice car, not like the kind my mother got. It was all new-looking and smelled good inside. It was such a treat for me, it was so long since I been in a car or even since I went outside the institution.

"We got a long way to go," Mrs. McKenna said.

"Could I touch your coat?"

"Sure you could touch it," she said. I put my fingers on it and rubbed, then I dig my fingers deep in the softness of it. It was softer than anything I ever felt, softer even than baby chickies.

There was snow on the ground and everything looked so pretty. I watched the houses go past, pretty houses that people lived in, that families lived in. I could see Christmas trees in the windows of some of them houses, Christmas trees all lit up like we use to have at my mother and daddy's. Some of the houses had decorations for Christmas all over, on the door, the windows, some even had lights outside. I never seen anything so beautiful. And there was a manger in front of one of the houses with Mary and Joseph and the Wise Men and the Baby Jesus.

"Oh, look, look!" I told Mrs. McKenna. "A manger!"

We went through some towns and, wouldn't you know it, them towns was all dressed up, too. The store windows and streets. Red and green lights and bells and Christmas trees and pictures of Santa Claus. Like the whole world was excited for Christmas.

I was looking out that window so hard I forgot where I was, forgot where I was going. All I could think of was, what a pretty world it is, the world is much prettier than the institution. I guess I been in that darn institution so long I forgot how pretty the outside world is.

Then we come to the country. Not too much houses there, just snow everywhere you look.

"Are we almost there?" I ask Mrs. McKenna.

"No, we still got a long time. We live up near your family. Our town is near to their town."

"Am I gonna see my mother and daddy?"

"I don't think so, not this time, but you're gonna have fun anyway."

Then Jeannie started fussing back there, kicking and showing she didn't want to be laying down no more. So Mrs. McKenna stopped the car and I got out and hop into the back seat with Jeannie, keep her busy. I didn't want to have her bothering Mrs. McKenna while she was driving.

Jeannie was feeling much better from having her teeths pulled, but she still looked funny. Different. I played with her fingers, I sing Christmas songs to her. Pretty soon she fell to sleep. She liked my singing, I think.

17

Oh, the McKennas got a lovely house, the kind of house I seen in magazine pictures. Rugs all over that place, you never seen so much rugs. You can't walk nowhere without having a rug under your feets, except the kitchen. We never had rugs at home and we sure as heck didn't have none in the institution.

They got a great big Christmas tree with so many lights it made me dizzy to look at them, all twinkling like stars. And Mr. McKenna was real nice. He said, "Hello, Winifred, so glad to meet you." He talked like that.

I said, "Hello, Mr. McKenna, so glad to meet you."

Jeannie got a little sister name of Prudence, she was pretty. Looked like Jeannie, but with teeths.

"This here's Prudence. Prudence, this here's Winifred," Mr. McKenna said. He was introducing us.

"Hello, Prudence, so glad to meet you," I said. But she

just grab onto her mother's coat, she was happy to see her, wouldn't leave go.

There was a wheeling chair in the living room and they took off Jeannie's coat and stuff and put her in the wheeling chair. She was just waking up. Must be she knew she was home, she yawned a couple times and looked around and got a real happy look on her little face.

"Go look under the tree, Winifred," Mrs. McKenna said. So I did and guess what. I seen two big packages, one said "Winifred" on it. My name, must be a present for me.

"Is this a present for me?"

"Sure is."

"Could I open it?"

"Of course you could." And they start in to open the other one; it was for Jeannie. They set on the floor and open it for her, so she could see what she got.

My present had such pretty paper all over it, red with pictures of Santa Claus, got a big red bow, too. I opened it real careful, didn't want to tear that pretty paper. Inside was a box, a big white box.

"Is there something inside this box?"

"Open it up and see, Winifred," Mrs. McKenna said. She was showing Jeannie the cute teddy bear that was in her present, fuzzy with shiny eyes. You could tell Jeannie loved it, she grabbed it and smiled real big so you could see her gums. Didn't want to leave go of that teddy bear.

So I opened the box. There was something in it, something soft and smooth and blue and white. Not a teddy bear. I took it out real careful. It looked like a dress to me. It looked like a new dress.

"Is it a dress?"

"Yes."

"Is it a new dress?"

"Yes."

"Oh thank you!" I said. Always I was wearing the stuff the institution give me; even at home I mostly had to wear

Wanda's stuff when it didn't fit her no more. I never got such a good present before.

"Could I put it on?"

"Let's go have lunch first. We been driving a long time and we didn't eat no lunch."

So we set in the kitchen, it was one of them sparkly kinds of kitchens, and when Mrs. McKenna opened the icebox to get out the tuna, I could see inside the icebox. It was stuffed near to busting, so full there wasn't even no room left.

"You sure got a lot of food," I told her.

Mr. McKenna and Prudence already ate, so Mrs. McKenna made tuna sandwiches for me and her. Not Jeannie, Jeannie had to have her food real soft and mashed, no sandwiches, 'cause she couldn't chew no more. Jeannie set near the table in her wheeling chair with her teddy bear, and me and Mrs. McKenna took turns feeding her the mashed-up tuna out of a bowl. She sure liked that tuna. So did I.

"Could I have seconds?" I ask. Mrs. McKenna didn't mind at all, she made me another tuna sandwich. I had two tuna sandwiches, two glasses of Ovaltine milk, two apples, and a lollipop. I shared my lollipop with Jeannie, let her take some licks, too.

Then off I go to try on my new dress. Mrs. McKenna took me upstairs where her bedroom was. Rugs there, too, even the upstairs got rugs all over the floor. And a great big mirror in her room, so big you could even see your feets in it.

She went out so I could put the dress on. I was glad she went out, I didn't want her to see the ratty bloomers I was wearing.

That dress felt so soft when I put it on, it felt soft and it was pretty like the kind of dresses Mrs. McKenna wore. It was all blue, got a white collar, white around the sleeves and got teeny white buttons down the front. They was awful hard to button, but I did get them buttoned. That dress felt so good on me. I felt pretty like Mrs. McKenna.

Then I went to the mirror and looked in. Looked and looked and looked, but it didn't matter how hard I looked, I didn't see nobody pretty, I didn't see nobody looked like Mrs. McKenna. Only thing I seen pretty was that dress. I looked like a dumb skinny old kid, I did. With dumb hair, my hair was all brown and short. And big ears, I got big ears sticking out.

The institution give me glasses 'cause I was having troubles seeing good, had to wear them glasses all the time. I seen good but I looked awful, my glasses looked like a little old lady's glasses. And my teeths, I didn't know that before—my teeths looked funny. Not all pokey-out like some of the other kids, but crooked. The teeths in front of my mouth didn't all point to the right way, some of them pointed to the wrong way. I never knew that about my teeths. We didn't have no mirror at the institution. The rest of me was skinny, long and skinny like an old giraffe.

I stood there and looked at all of me. I didn't look like Mrs. McKenna. I looked like one of them retarded kids.

I set down on the bed in my brand new dress. I wasn't gonna come out of that room, didn't want no one in the world to look at me.

Then I hear "bump, bump" on the door.

"Winifred?" It was Mrs. McKenna.

"What, Mrs. McKenna?"

"Could I come in?"

"Okay."

She come in and seen me setting on her bed looking gloomy as could be.

"What's the matter? Don't you like the dress?"

"Mrs. McKenna, I seen in the mirror. The dress is pretty but I'm not pretty. I don't even look like you at all."

"Oh, Winifred," Mrs. McKenna said, real nice. "You look real good. And you got a lovely smile, did you know that? When you smile your whole face looks pretty, when you smile your whole face lights up."

"My whole face lights up?"

"Sure does. And you look pretty in that dress, you look real nice in blue."

"But my hair's too short. It makes me look retarded. People are gonna think I'm retarded."

"Winifred, my sister got short hair in Florida, short hair almost like you got. She's real pretty, she looks pretty with her hair like that. And so do you. Now come downstairs so Mr. McKenna could see you in your new dress."

I think Mrs. McKenna was just trying to be kind to me, saying all them things.

I stayed at the McKennas' a couple days. I really liked it there. Mrs. McKenna took me to town, took me to see all the stores. Oh, they was beautiful, full of Christmas, and so many pretty things I could never get my full of just looking at all them things. Even the people in the stores was nice-looking. I like the way outside people look, they don't look like institution people. I had such fun watching everyone, seeing what lovely clothes they got on, seeing what kind of hair. Only thing, you worry that people will know where you come from, you worry that maybe they might find out you come from an institution. That's something you don't want nobody to know. You want people to think you're just like everyone else.

Mrs. McKenna give me a dollar, took me to the Woolworth store. Said I could buy anything I want. Did I ever have a hard time picking, seemed like they got everything in the whole world at Woolworth's. Didn't know what to look at first.

I thought, hmmmm, maybe jacks, the game of jacks with the ball. Then I seen the wind-up toys, like a little monkey and you wind it up and it goes all by itself. I kept winding it up, I was laughing and laughing, it was so fun to watch it go. The store lady told me to stop, said you're not allowed to wind things up. Anyway, I didn't want to buy that monkey, didn't like the look it got on the face.

There was all kinds of candy. I thought maybe I could get

me some candy to eat such as gumdrops or chocolate babies. But after you eat it up, you're not gonna have nothing left. Lipsticks. Lipsticks in all pretty colors. Uh-uh. They wouldn't never let me wear lipstick at the institution, so what's the use?

Mrs. McKenna started getting tired 'cause I was taking so long, said, "Come on, Winifred, you gotta hurry now." She left Jeannie and Prudence with Mr. McKenna and they must be waiting on us.

"Oh, look at all the jewelry, Mrs. McKenna!" Rings, necklaces, bracelets, and pins. I told her, "I want a ring!" But it was too hard to pick out which color—the rings got all colors of jewels—so Mrs. McKenna had to help me choose. She picked out a ring with a great big red jewel, said she thought that was the best one. I paid for it with my dollar and the lady give me some of my money back. She start to put the ring in a bag but I said, "No, no, I want to wear it right now."

All the way home I didn't look at the stores or the houses, just looked at my finger wearing that shiny red ring. The jewel was sparkly, it sparkled like the lights on the McKennas' Christmas tree.

I was a big help to Mrs. McKenna while I was there. Helped with Jeannie. Like feed her, she mostly had to eat baby food. Helped change her diapers. And when she cried I make funny faces at her, or do the sounds Mrs. Knopf was always showing me, my speech practices. That made Jeannie laugh. Sometimes she tried to copy me.

Jeannie had to take medicine all the time. She didn't like it, but I held her on my lap. She was getting big—twelve years old, almost too big to set on your lap—but I could hold her and Mrs. McKenna put the spoon in her mouth. Then always she made a silly face when she taste that medicine, a bad face.

Also, I play with Prudence. She was a real sweet kid. She got a big sled for her Christmas present and we dress up warm and go out in the yard and I pull her on the sled. We even made a snowmans. Big ball of snow for a tummy, little ball of snow for a head. It was easy as pies. Wasn't no face, but Mr. McKenna give us an old cap to go on the head. Then, oh boy, did that snowmans ever look real. When we get cold, in the house we come, and Mrs. McKenna give us cocoa and we played with my new cards. Mrs. McKenna showed us how to do it. I really liked Prudence, she was so little and pretty. Looked just like Jeannie when she first come to the institution.

When we have our lunch or supper, Mrs. McKenna all the time give me seconds. And after supper, dessert time, always time for dessert after supper. Such as chocolate cake, baked apples, yummy things like that. If I want a little snack before bedtime I just say, "Mrs. McKenna, could I have a little snack?" And she'd say, "Help yourself, Winifred." That means you could go get something to eat. So off I skip to the kitchen and get me some milk and cookies or some cake, maybe a couple bananas—get some milk, too, to wash it all down. I found it such fun to help myself.

I could of stayed at the McKennas' house forever and ever.

18

I was feeling real blue. It's hard to go back to an institution when you been in freedom a couple days. You could say I was being grumpy and cranky. Could be 'cause I wasn't getting any sleep when I first come back. I was use to quiet at the McKennas' house. Sometimes Jeannie cried in the night, but that wasn't nothing like the screams and fits in the institution. Took me awhile to get use to it again.

Minnie wasn't in Children's Cottage no more, neither

was Estelle Sampson. 'Cause when you're done school, you get put in one of the grown-up buildings. Minnie was the worse one with the fits, but there was a new girl name Annie, she was almost as bad.

I laid there all the first night I was back, just like when I first come to the institution when I was six years old. I laid there waiting for the fits. Ruby Rose and Dolly was crying in their sleep with nightmares. Then Josephine started in screaming and making such a racket Miss Busby had to run in, wake her up, get her out of that dream so she wouldn't wake the other kids.

And all the night I'm laying there thinking about the outside world, thinking about the McKennas' house and all the rugs they got on the floors, and the stores full of pretty people with pretty hair and all them nice clothes. And I'm thinking, why can't I be in the outside world, too?

Mrs. Spencer threw my dress on the floor. It was the blue dress the McKennas give me. Just 'cause I said, "I don't want to wear that. I wore it yesterday and it's not clean no more."

"Nobody asked you," Mrs. Spencer said.

"Well, I'm not going around smelling. I want my dress washed."

"Put that darn dress on!" Only she didn't say "darn."

"No!"

What she done next was terrible. She called for a straitjacket. I never been in a straitjacket before, but I seen girls get put in them. That's how they have to do to girls who get really disturbed, keep them tied in a straitjacket till they come to their senses, act normal. But they got to get permission from Mrs. Treadwell to do it. Mrs. Spencer didn't get permission. She just told the cleaning lady to hurry up get her a straitjacket for Winifred.

I got scared, didn't know what the heck she was doing. I yelled, "I don't wanna go in a straitjacket!" But she just told me to be still, got the cleaning lady to help hold me while she tied me up in that thing. I was hollering and yowling.

"Shut up!" she said. Some of the kids start coming in to see what all the racket was about. Took one look and run right out again.

Mrs. Spencer wasn't suppose to be doing what she was doing. I bet she didn't want Mrs. Treadwell to know, I bet that's why she wanted me to shut up. But I wouldn't shut up. How can you shut up when you're hysterical?

She left me there hollering, come back in a minute with a pillowcase. The pillowcase was all wet. She said, "Are you gonna shut up now, Winifred, or do I gotta shut you up with this?"

I called, "Help! Help!"

She come at me with that pillowcase, she got fire in her face. My heart was beating like it was gonna bust out. I tried to fight and kick with my feets, but you can't do too much when you're tied up in a straitjacket. She pushed that thing down over my head, over my face, that wet pillowcase. It felt awful, it felt cold, I couldn't see nothing. Couldn't hardly breathe. She thought that would shut me up, but it just made me get more hysterical.

I heard people coming and I start to pass out. Couldn't get enough air, could hardly get air at all inside that thing. I felt dizzy and I heard someone call out to me, call my name. I think it was Mrs. Drake. I said, "Who?" and then I went into unconscious, I don't remember nothing. Lucy told me they had to cut the straitjacket off me, cut the pillowcase off me, 'cause Mrs. Spencer tied it around my neck with a laundry rope. Lucy seen all the fussing over me, she told me they come with a stretcher and all the kids watched me going out on the stretcher, going to the hospital. But I don't remember nothing.

When I woke up it was dark and the nurse that was setting next to me called out, "She come out of it." Things was all bleary and I seen the nurse and I said, "Oh, where am I?"

Then everything went clear and I remembered. I thought I was still in the pillowcase and I screamed and screamed. I felt my nightie getting all wet, then the bed felt wet, 'cause while I was screaming I messed the bed. But I couldn't help it, I didn't know what I was doing. I was so disturbed. They give me a needle and I fell to sleep again even in my wet nightie.

When I open my eyes again it was daytime. Mrs. Treadwell come and Mr. Buckholz was with her.

"How did I get here, how did I get to the hospital?"

"We want you to answer some questions, Winifred," Mr. Buckholz said.

"Why did Mrs. Spencer put that pillowcase on your head, put that straitjacket on you?" Mrs. Treadwell ask me.

"'Cause I wouldn't put my dress on."

"Why wouldn't you put your dress on?"

"'Cause it was dirty, 'cause I wanted it to be washed."

I was glad to tell them what happened, I was glad to tell on Mrs. Spencer. She should never did what she did, especially with a wet pillowcase on the head.

I laid in that hospital a couple days. Sometimes I would get upset all over again and cry and they have to come give me some calm medicine. I was so disturbed, in such a state, couldn't even eat my food.

Once I heard the nurse tell someone, "Out! Winifred's not allowed to have no visitors." She was talking to Mrs. Spencer. I could see them in the hall. I could have visitors, but not her. I never liked Mrs. Spencer, but after she done that thing I despise her. They suspended her for five days, she's lucky they didn't fire her. And she was suppose to be a Catholic. But she got her day. God took care of her. She died in the summer with a heart attack.

For a long time after that, I couldn't use a pillow.

The last day I was in the hospital the nurse come in.

"Winifred, you got company."

Guess who. Gladys! I was so thrilled to see Gladys, she

never come to see me before that. Oh, she looked good to me. She said, "How you doing, Winnie?"

"Fine, I'm fine, I'm so glad you come to see me!"

"Look what I got for you," she said, and she opened up her pocketbook and took out a little box of gingersnaps. "Do you still like gingersnaps?"

"Oh boy, I sure do!"

"I heard what happened to you. What a terrible thing for someone to do." But I didn't even answer, I was eating my gingersnaps. They tasted so good, put me in mind of when I was little and she was always bringing me gingersnaps at home.

"How's my mother and daddy?" I ask her after I ate a whole bunch of gingersnaps.

"They're okay. Miriam got married at Thanksgiving. Now she lives in town near where I live."

"How come nobody ever comes to see me?" I ask her. "Nobody even writes, daddy don't even write no more."

"Well, must be he's so busy with the chickens. But I got a car now and I'll come see you again."

"Would you take me to a restaurant next time you come? 'Cause I never been in a restaurant."

"Sure, Winnie, sure I will."

"Oh goody!" I said, and I ate some more gingersnaps.

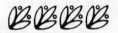

SPRING
1947

19

I set in the yard with Jeannie and the other low-grades watching the springtime coming in. The flowers was just starting and the robins was humming and the sun was shining warm on us. Even the low-grades seemed happy. In the springtime everything is so beautiful, it makes me think of God more.

Also, when the weather comes warm, it means I could see Jeannie a lot. I don't get to see her much in cold weather, mostly I could only see her when we're all outside. I miss Jeannie in winter, I miss looking out for her. You could say she's like my little sister. I treat her like a princess and give her everything, even to love.

On warm days I ask Mrs. Drake or Miss Emmett could I go over and see Jeannie? Most times they say yes, yes, Winifred, you could go. Oh, it makes my heart feel good to see her. She's not so pretty no more 'cause after she lost her teeths her mouth went all funny looking. But she still got them big blue eyes and pretty curls, blonde hair just like her mother got. And always Jeannie is happy to see me coming. You could say it makes me feel good, real good, that there is someone happy to see me coming.

"Look at the flower, Jeannie," I said, and I pull a little yellow flower up for her, held it under her chin to see if she likes butter. She wasn't in her wheeling chair, she was laying on a big mat on the grass with another low-grade. "Oh, Jeannie, you like butter."

But Jeannie just laid there on her mat. Not playing or waving her cute little hands or laughing. She was just watching me and watching the flower with them big eyes. I look at her real close. Her eyes didn't look right.

"Mrs. Paretti, Mrs. Paretti," I called, "Jeannie don't look right."

Mrs. Paretti was setting on the grass under a tree talking to another attendant, looked like she didn't want to be bothered. "Jeannie's okay," she said, and just went on talking.

"No, she's not," I said. "Mrs. Paretti, Mrs. Paretti, Jeannie don't look right."

Mrs. Paretti got up with a growly look on the face. She come over, said, "Looks okay to me. Could be she just wants her nap."

"No, Mrs. Paretti, her eyes look funny and she's just laying there. Not doing nothing, No kicking, no laughing." The low-grades is always doing something, laughing or crying, they're not quiet much. Only if they're sleeping. "Maybe she's sick, Mrs. Paretti."

Mrs. Paretti set down next to Jeannie and feel of her head. "Well," she said, "she does feel kind of warm." So I help her lift Jeannie back in her wheeling chair. It wasn't too easy to lift Jeannie no more 'cause she was getting big.

"I better take her inside."

"Oh, Mrs. Paretti, could I come?"

"No, Winifred, you go back to your own building."

20

The girls was making Easter hats when I come back. Miss West—she's the lady use to help us make scrapbooks, she was showing them how. They was all setting down in the playroom with paper plates and paper flowers.

"Set down, Winifred, so I could show you how to make an Easter hat," Miss West told me. She give me a paper plate, showed me how to cut out the middle so it goes over my head. Then I got to pick out what color flowers. I pick blue and red ones and I glue them real careful all over the hat and I put it on my head. Then I go all around the playroom with that hat on my head, walking like I'm a real fine lady.

Ruby Rose said, "Look at my hat!" She got yellow flowers on hers. All them hats was so pretty.

Us older kids had to help the ones who can't cut, we help them cut the plates so they go onto their heads right. But some of the kids got them real big heads, too hard to make the paper plates fit. So Miss West had to do it, cut great big holes for the ones with great big heads.

Then we all put our hats away on the top shelf real neat, so they don't get messed. 'Cause when Easter comes, we make a parade all around the institution, show off our hats what we made. Then we go to church in the Assembly Hall, we wear our pretty hats to church. Easter is my favorite holiday. That's when Our Lord rose from the dead.

All the time I was doing the hats, I was wondering about Jeannie, that's all I could think of, Jeannie. So when we was done, I ask Miss Emmett could I go back over to Forest, see if Jeannie's sick or not sick.

"No, Winifred, you got to eat your supper soon."

"I don't want any darn supper," I said, real nasty. Miss Emmett looked like she might get mean, so I thought, well, maybe I better eat my supper.

After supper I tried Mrs. Drake. "Mrs. Drake, could I go over to Forest? I think Jeannie's sick."

"It's too late, you can't go out after supper. Go down to the playroom."

"Please, Mrs. Drake. 'Cause I promised Jeannie's mother I'd help look out for her."

"No, Winifred!"

I stomp into the playroom, set down at one of the tables, act real grumpy. Two of the littler girls was running around making noises. I growled, "Shut up, will you?" All them noises was getting on my nerves, making me nervous. 'Cause I was worried about Jeannie.

So I wait till we was all in bed and most of the kids was asleep, then I tippytoe out like I'm going to the bathroom. Miss Busby and Mrs. O'Brien didn't even see me going. Foxy old Winifred.

Real quick I run out of the building and over to Forest. I was wearing my nightie, that's all I got on me, nothing on my feets. It was cold, my feets was cold, and it hurt to run on the driveway in just my feets. I run up the steps into Forest Building, I must of looked a sight, and one of the attendants—she didn't know me 'cause she was a night attendant—she said, "Who are you?"

"How's Jeannie?" I said. "How's Jeannie McKenna?"

"You're not suppose to be here, you're suppose to be in bed."

"I just want to see Jeannie, find out if she's okay."

"You're not allowed up there," she said in a snarly way.

"You better let me up there," I said back in a snarly way, "'cause I'm like a sister to Jeannie and Jeannie's like a sister to me, and I wanna see how she's doing."

When I said that, the attendant got a look on her face, looked like she might be scared. Could be she thought I was one of them real disturbed ones. She just turn around and walk away from me. Maybe she figured she better not get me mad.

Upstairs I run, straight to the room where Jeannie lived. I could hear all them low-grades fussing and crying. Jeannie was laying in her crib, but she wasn't asleep. Some of the lights was on and I could see her face looked all pink and her eyes was shiny like they was when we was outside. She wasn't crying, she wasn't laughing, wasn't doing nothing, just once in awhile there come a little cough. Didn't smell too good, neither, I could see her diaper needed changing. But I didn't mind the smell, her smell didn't bother me none.

"Hi Jeannie, look who's here. It's me, Winifred."

Jeannie turned her head a little and just looked at me, but she didn't look happy to see me. Looked like she just didn't care about nothing. I felt scared, she looked so bad.

I stood by her crib and rubbed her head and her tummy like I always done for her. She loved her head and tummy to get rubbed. And I sang, I sang some church songs and "Silent Night." But while I'm singing, I hear someone coming behind me. Miss Busby.

"Winifred, what the heck are you doing over here?"

"Jeannie's sick," I said. "I had to come see her." I was glad it was Miss Busby come after me and not Mrs. O'Brien. Mrs. O'Brien wasn't always too kind.

"You know you got no rights to run out of the building at night without telling no one, especially in your nightie and barefeets."

"But I was worried about Jeannie. I promised her mother I'd look out for her, but no one would let me come see her. I'm like Jeannie's sister and Jeannie's like my sister."

Miss Busby went and talked to one of the Forest attendants who was standing by the door watching me. Then she come back.

"Jeannie's got a big temperature, but the attendants is giving her medicine to help her get better. She's getting good care, so don't worry about her. Now you come back with me and go to bed."

Was I surprised she wasn't mad. Must be she knew how worried I was about Jeannie. And when I was in bed she was telling Mrs. O'Brien, "I know Winifred run out of the building in the middle of the night, but I'm not gonna punish her. She was worried about a sick kid, she was worried about Jeannie McKenna. She's like a sister to Jeannie and Jeannie's like a sister to her."

21

"I gotta go see Jeannie," I told Mrs. Drake soon as I got my bath and put my clothes on. She said okay, didn't even tell me I had to get my breakfast first, 'cause it wasn't a school day.

Boy, did I run to Forest. In the hall right away I seen Mrs. Paretti. "How's Jeannie, Mrs. Paretti? Could I go up there?"

"They just took Jeannie to the hospital, Winifred."

"The hospital? Why is she in the hospital?"

"She got pneumonia," she told me.

I wanted to run right over to the hospital. But I couldn't. They wouldn't of let me in, we wasn't allowed to visit at the hospital.

I went back to Children's Cottage. All I could think of was, suppose Jeannie was gonna die, suppose she died on me. No more Jeannie. No more going to visit Jeannie. No more someone happy to see me coming.

"Mrs. Drake, Jeannie's in the hospital. She got pneumonia." The tears start to come, I couldn't help it. "Mrs. Drake, maybe she's gonna die."

Mrs. Drake was real nice sometimes, she didn't try to make me eat my breakfast. She could tell I was all worked up, she could see I was upset about Jeannie. "Don't worry," she said. "They got good medicine and good doctors at the hospital. Jeannie's gonna be okay."

"But can't I see her? I promised her mother I'd look out for her. Maybe she's scared 'cause she don't know no one in the hospital, maybe she'll feel better if she sees me."

"You're not allowed to visit in the hospital," Mrs. Drake said. "Now stop your crying. Jeannie's gonna get better soon."

But I couldn't stop. Just 'cause someone tells you to stop

your crying don't mean you could do it. I went into the playroom, set at one of the little tables. The cleaning lady was in there. She was ironing.

"What's wrong with you, child, why you crying?" she ask me. She called all the kids "child."

I told her, "I'm crying 'cause my friend is sick."

I wanted to go to the hospital to see Jeannie. But the only way I could get in the hospital was if I was sick, too. Like chicken poxes. Or polio. Ruby Rose got polio last year, or maybe it was the year before last year, and she stayed a long time in the hospital. Now she got a bad leg with a brace on it. I didn't want to get polio.

Also could go to the hospital if you get hurt. Like a broken bone. Maybe I could get a broken bone. When the cleaning lady went upstairs I run over, grab up the iron, let that iron go on my foot.

"Help!" I called, "help, help, help!" and I start in yelling and hollering. It hurt, boy, did that iron hurt me when it hit my foot. I didn't think it would hurt so bad. I start to cry and I keep calling "Help, help!" and the cleaning lady run back down, got her arms full of dresses.

"What happened?" she said, then she run upstairs again and come back with Miss Emmett.

I was crying so hard, it hurt me so much, I couldn't even tell them what happened. Miss Emmett figured it out though, she seen the iron on the floor near to my foot. She made me set down and she took my shoe and sock off to see what my foot looked like. It looked bad, it did, all red.

"Wiggle your toes, Winifred. Could you wiggle your toes?" Mrs. Drake asked. I guess she come down when she heard all the racket.

"I can't, I can't, I can't wiggle my toes."

"She can't wiggle her toes," Mrs. Drake said.

"See if she could walk," Miss Emmett said. So they stand me up and try to make me walk, but I can't. My foot hurt too much.

"No, no," I yowled, "I can't walk, oh, oh, it hurts!"

They got a wheeling chair to take me to the hospital. But my foot hurt so much from that darn iron and I was hollering so much, I wasn't even thinking about Jeannie no more. You could even say I forgot about her. All I could think of was my foot, how bad my foot hurt. My big toe was starting to get all swelled up, too.

They took X-ray pictures of it and then I had to set with the nurse until they could find out about my foot, if it was broke or not broke. She was a nice nurse, a pretty nurse, she helped take care of me when I was in the hospital with a pillowcase on the head. I remembered her and she remembered me. She was joking with me, made me laugh, while we was waiting to find out about my foot.

The doctor come out and he said to the nurse, "It's broke. She broke it."

"My foot is broke?" I was feeling better. I was thinking about Jeannie again, that maybe I could ask them real nice to put me in the bed near to Jeannie.

"No, Winifred, your toe is broke."

"So I gotta stay in the hospital and get a cast?"

"No," he told me, "you don't need no cast for a broken toe and you don't need to stay in the hospital. You just got to wear a soft slipper for a long time and not walk around too much, keep off your feets."

"But why can't I be in the hospital?"

"Why do you want to be in the hospital?"

"'Cause of Jeannie, I want to be with Jeannie McKenna. I promised her mother I'd look after her."

The doctor give the nurse a look, then he ask me, "Did you let that iron go on your foot? Did you do that to yourself?"

"Yes," I said.

22

They made me stay inside two weeks, that was my punishment. Couldn't go out nowhere, just set around all the darn day, nothing to do. Couldn't walk much, anyway.

I missed the Easter parade. It was raining a little, the drippy kind of raining, but they had the parade anyway 'cause they didn't want to disappoint the girls. They was in such a dither, all looking forward to it.

I set and watched it from the window. All the grown-up girls come marching by in their Easter hats, marching and dancing up the driveway. They was holding hands and some was even singing. You could tell they was so proud of theirselfs and their Easter hats which they made, they didn't even care about the rain. But I could see the rain was messing up them hats.

Then come the kids, the kids from Children's Cottage. The ones in wheeling chairs was there, even a couple of the real retarded kids was there. They was wearing hats somebody made for them, they wasn't smart enough to make their own. Ruby Rose's hat was hanging down a little 'cause it was getting wet. And the yellow flowers was ruined, the yellow flowers looked like squashy wet stuff. But she kept marching along like she didn't care, or maybe she didn't know her Easter hat was going all to pieces in the rain. She had a big smile on her face like she was feeling beautiful.

If I set at the window near to Dolly's bed, I could see Jeannie out in the yard sometimes. She looked okay far as I could tell, just a little skinny. I was glad. But I couldn't go see her, I was still being punished.

Mrs. Knopf come to see me on her way to school. That made me feel good, showed she cared about me. She got a book with her.

"How's your toe, Winifred?"

"Okay, Mrs. Knopf."

"That wasn't a good thing to do, let an iron go on your toe."

"I know, Mrs. Knopf, I learned my lesson. I'm not gonna do it never again."

She give me the book she was carrying. She told me, "This here's for you to read while you're getting better. Bring it back to school when you come."

"But I can't read yet, Mrs. Knopf. Only some words. I can't read books."

"Try it," she said.

I set on my bed after she left and looked at the book. It had lots of pictures in it, pretty pictures, and lots of stories. Well, I thought, let's see if I could read it.

I start in to read and guess what, I kept going. It was coming easy. Told about these little kids—they was Dick and Jane and Sally—and all the adventures they get in. And I'm just going along, went right through two stories, and then I stop and say, wait a minute, I'm *reading*.

"Mrs. Drake! Miss Emmett! Mrs. Drake! Miss Emmett! I could read, I could read, I could read!" I hop out into the hall. There was Mrs. Drake tying shoes for one of the kids.

"Winifred, what's going on?"

"Listen, Mrs. Drake, listen!" And I read the first story to her, told about Sally found a red ball and she played a game with the red ball.

"Oh, Winifred, that's real nice," she said.

"Miss Emmett, Miss Emmett," I holler, and I hop downstairs. Miss Emmett was setting in the dining room getting her breakfast. She looked at me coming, she look at me like, what's Winifred up to now? But I just set down right next to her and I read the story about the kids' dog runs away and can't find that dog no place. Miss Emmett told me when I was done, "Oh, you read that story real good."

I was all in a dither, didn't know what to do next. I went to the kitchen ladies and read them a story, too. They was washing up the dishes, but they stop to listen to me, tell me how nice I read. The cleaning lady was in the bathroom, she was mopping up the floor. She let me read two stories to her, she told me, "Oh, what good stories. Them stories is better than what I heard on the radio last night."

Then I hop back up to the dorm and set on my bed and read some more. I really liked them stories. Told about Jane having a party, and told about the little cat they got and the nice-looking mother and daddy. The daddy plays with them and the mother bakes cookies. I like best when I come to the part where they go visit a farm, all about the animals and them kids played in the barn with the chickens, the cows and the horses. That was my favorite part. It give me such joy to read, like the book was talking to me and I could hear what it was saying.

When I seen the kids coming back from school, I yell out the window, didn't even wait till they got in the building, "I could read, I could read!"

And I set down with Ruby Rose while we was waiting for lunch, and some of the little kids set down too, and I read to them all about the farm and the animals.

"Oh, that's a good story," Gloria said. "Would you read to us another story?"

"Who wants to hear them dumb old stories?" Ruby Rose said. I bet she wished she could read.

So I read another story to Gloria and Dolly and Bonnie— oh, I felt so proud and smart—and then it was time for lunch. And I bring that book down with me to lunch and even to supper, nobody could of got that book out of my hands, I just like to see anybody try.

When I hit a hard word, I show it to Mrs. Drake or Miss Emmett, get them to tell me the word. Or sometimes I just skip that word, go on to the next word that I could understand. By the time bedtime come, I read that whole darn book. Before I went to sleep I put the book under my bed, make sure I could find it right away in the morning.

Next day I read the book again, every single story. When

somebody come and try to talk to me or tease me I just said, "Don't bother me, I'm reading a book." And I didn't care that I was being punished, didn't care that I couldn't go out, didn't even care about my foot hurting me. 'Cause when I read them stories, it put my mind someplace else that I wish to be, instead of where I am.

23

I got a letter from Gladys, had to ask Miss Emmett to read it for me 'cause it was in script. Miss Emmett read that Gladys was coming to see me next time it was visiting day!

I couldn't wait until visiting day. I didn't see Gladys in such a long time, not since I been in the hospital. But she sent me a present for Christmas, beautiful red mittens, also a birthday card when my birthday come.

I told everybody, "Guess what, my sister Gladys is coming to see me. I'm getting company." I was so proud.

"So what, so what if you're getting company?" Ruby Rose growled. She didn't have no company in a long time, her mother didn't come in years, or maybe she died.

I woke up before anyone else on visiting day, hop out of bed, get my bath, get dressed, get my breakfast and set out in the yard to wait. Oh, I felt so important, I set on one of the swings like a queen. I was waiting for my sister to come.

"Look at Winifred," Annie said, "she thinks she's so smart, just setting there waiting for her sister."

"So what, at least someone's coming to visit me. I bet no one's coming to visit you."

"Maybe Winifred don't even have a sister," Ruby Rose said. I could tell she wanted to fight with me, I could tell she was being jealous. But I thought, nope, I better not fight. I didn't want Gladys to come and see me right in the middle of socking somebody.

Then a car drove up. It wasn't Gladys, it was Annie's family, Annie's mother and daddy. Annie give me a ratty look, then she run to meet them.

"So what!" I yelled. "You don't have a sister!"

I set there on the swing all morning. A couple of the little girls got company, their families come and take them away in their cars and they was all excited and squealing. I started to worry. Could be Miss Emmett read that letter wrong, could be what Gladys wrote was that she wasn't coming to see me next visiting day. Or could be Gladys forgot.

Then I seen her. I seen a green car coming slow up the driveway and right away I seen that red hair, that red hair that Gladys got, and I said to myself, oh boy, must be that's Gladys!

I wanted to run to the car, but I couldn't. Still got my bad toe, had to wear a slipper on my foot that got the front cut so my toes could stick out in the air.

I hollered, "Gladys, Gladys, here I am, Gladys!"

She stop the car out front, didn't even go to the parking lot, she got out and come straight into the yard. Give me a big hug right in front of all the other kids. I give her a big hug, too. She had perfume on.

"Oh, Winnie, it's so good to see you," she said when we was done with hugging.

"So why didn't you come in such a long time if it's so good to see me?"

" 'Cause I'm working in a factory now, and factory work keeps you pretty busy."

"Did you bring me gingersnaps?"

"No, I didn't bring you no gingersnaps, but I thought we could go to a restaurant 'cause you told me you wanted to go to a restaurant last time I seen you."

"Oh, goody, goody!"

Gladys had to go inside first, tell Mrs. Treadwell she come to take Winifred out. When we was going to the car she seen me walking funny, she seen the slipper I got on my foot.

"What happened to your foot?"

I was ashamed to tell her I done it to myself. "Oh, nothing," I said, "just an iron that dropped down on it."

What a thrill to be in a restaurant. It was a beautiful restaurant, too, got a jukebox that played music just like the one we got in the canteen. We set at a table, the table got a red cloth on it, a table cloth. Real fancy. And got a bottle of sugar and ketchup and some salt and pepper, in case you need them things when you're eating. A lady come, she was wearing a red dress and an apron. She give us each a big paper. I said, "What's this?"

"It's a menu," Gladys said. "Tells what the restaurant has for eating."

I set there and looked at my menu just like Gladys was looking at her menu. It was too hard for me to read, but I didn't want the lady to know that. She might think I was from the institution.

"I'm gonna have the roast chicken, Winnie. What are you gonna have?"

"Oh, that's what I want, I want the roast chicken too."

So Gladys told the lady we want the roast chicken and the lady wrote it down on a tablet, wrote down what Gladys said. Then she ask me did I want potatoes. I said yes, I sure did want potatoes, and she ask me did I want the french frieds or the baked. I couldn't make up my mind. I said, "Couldn't I have them both, the french frieds and the baked?" Gladys said I could only have one, I had to choose, so I choosed the french frieds. Then we had to choose corn or stringbeans, you couldn't eat both of them. Gladys choosed the corn, so I did, too. Last of all, you got to choose what to drink. Right away I said, "Root beer, give me root beer!" 'cause I had root beer when I was at the McKennas' and I think root beer is delicious.

That lady was so darn polite, even to calling me "Miss"

when she was asking me the questions. That made me feel important.

Then we had to just set while they was cooking our food. There was a mother and daddy at a table near to us, got two little kids with them. They was so cute, wiggling around and laughing, couldn't set still. There was some ladies at another table eating and talking away, looked to be having a good time, and there was a pretty lady setting with a man. She had beautiful long hair, lipstick and makeup on her face. She kept putting money in the jukebox, so everybody could listen to the music. I think our jukebox in the canteen is a better jukebox. You don't need to put no money in to hear the music.

I started humming, I knew the song that was playing, and Gladys said, "Don't do that, Winnie, don't hum real loud. Everyone is gonna look at you." She was right, too. The mother and the daddy was looking at me. I shut up real quick. I didn't want no one to look at me, didn't want no one to think I was different.

"Listen, Winnie, I got something to tell you," Gladys said. "You know what? I got married."

"Oh, that's good. That's nice."

"I got married last summer. To a real sweet man, his name is Clayton."

"Could you bring Clayton to visit me, too?"

"Well, I don't know. He has to drive a truck all the time, he don't get much days off."

"How's my mother? How's my daddy?"

"They're fine, everybody is fine. Said to say hello to you."

I was real hungry. They sure was taking their time cooking our food for us, but I guess it takes a long time 'cause they gotta cook the other people's food, too. And Gladys said you can't get up and walk around in a restaurant, neither. You just set there and wait your turn to get your food cooked.

Gladys and me talked. I told her about school, I told her I learned to read. She praised me, said I was doing real fine.

"Look, look, here comes the lady with the roast chicken!" I hollered. Oh boy, did that roast chicken ever smell good. I started to gobble it up the minute that lady put my plate down.

"You must of been real hungry," she said.

I didn't even answer her, got my mouth stuffed up with that chicken already. She went away and come back with my root beer, give me a great big glass, even with a straw to drink from. They sure got good food in that restaurant, better than the institution, and you get more of it, too. Lots of chicken, lots of french frieds, lots of corn.

"Winnie, you're eating the bone," Gladys said.

"The bone? What bone? I don't see no bone." It was soft, it was so soft I didn't even know it was the bone. I guess I was gobbling too fast to see it go by.

"Slow down, Winnie, slow down," Gladys said, but she was laughing, she wasn't mad at me. She looked so pretty when she laughed. I tried to eat slow like Gladys was eating slow, but it was hard. That food tasted so good. And I ate every bit of it, cleaned my plate.

"I thought she was gonna eat the picture off that plate," the lady told Gladys. She took up my plate and went to get Gladys's plate. I wiped all the chicken off my face real careful with my napkin. I learned them manners at the McKennas'. That's how Mrs. McKenna does when she eats.

"You got a good restaurant here," I told the lady. "You got real good food."

"Thank you," she said. She was real nice; you could tell she was a friendly lady.

Then come dessert time. Got to choose again. It was hard to decide. Hmmmmmm, should I have the chocolate pudding or jello or blueberry pie or maybe the cherry pie or I could even have ice cream.

"Couldn't I pick two things?" I ask Gladys, "couldn't I pick two things for dessert?"

"Sure, Winnie, sure you could pick two things."

Gladys had to help me, it was too hard. All them goodies. I had cherry pie and chocolate pudding. Gladys just had
coffee and she poured sugar in her coffee from the bottle.

I ate all my cherry pie, I ate all my chocolate pudding.
Gladys had to laugh to see me eat so much.

"I hope you'll come back soon," I told Gladys when we
was in the car.

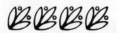

AUTUMN
1952

24

Being in an institution is like being away at college. You're learning. The smarter girls say, "I'm not here 'cause I'm retarded, I'm here to learn stuff." We have friends and ladies here to help us, also special classes for the kids who can't talk or hear too good.

The institution is real pretty in the summer and fall. They keep it nice, the trees and bushes and grass. It sure looks like a college to me.

I was doing good in school. We had spelling tests and I could do them, I sound out my letters and I got good grades. Every morning we do our geography. I had lots of troubles with arithmetic, though. Learned to carry my numbers but didn't know my times tables. Too hard to remember all that stuff. Sometimes I ask if I could have my arithmetic workbook to take out to do so I could practice. The answers I didn't know I just wait till next day, then I get Mrs. Knopf to help me with the pages that is giving me troubles.

Mrs. Knopf even give me a piece to say in front of the whole class. I had to learn all the words, and I did learn all the words. It was about in summer when you go to bed you could still hear the birds, in winter I get up at night and dress by candlelight. Isn't that something, it's still up there in my brain.

I was working so hard Mrs. Knopf put me in the highest group. I was doing fourth-grade work in everything but arithmetic. Especially reading and writing. That was my best thing. Reading and writing was my hobby ever since I learn to read and write.

Once Mrs. Knopf told us to write a story about Election Day. So the next day the other girls turn their papers in. Mrs. Knopf said, "Winifred, where's your paper?"

"It's not done yet, Mrs. Knopf." I was getting newspapers from the attendants. Nibby-nose Winifred kept looking in a whole lot of newspapers and everything I could find about Election Day I copy into my story. I was using the newspapers to get information. Real smart.

Pretty soon one morning I come to school and hand my paper in. Was Mrs. Knopf surprised! She said mine was the longest story, got the most information, said I done real good and she give me a gold star.

Also I was reading all the time. I wanted books so bad I always look in the school library for books that I could read. Such as science and geography and fairy tales. I find it such fun to read. When I read I make believe; I put my mind into different cities that I wish I could go to in person. Such as France, Hawaii and Florida, all them places I wished I could go to. But I know you have to ride in a plane to get there and I never been in a plane. I would be real nervous until I get back to the ground again. I wonder can you walk around in a plane? I think that could make the plane tip over.

I always had a book to take home with me after school 'cause I knew reading would prove I was learning fast.

Mrs. Knopf was still helping me with my speech when she got time, and sometimes I got to the regular speech teacher, Mrs. Durand. She holds up cards with sounds on them and we kids got to say the sounds over and over. The hardest for me was the "w" and the "th" sound. We done exercises with our lips, with our mouths too. I try very hard. My speech was getting better, I could tell. 'Cause when I was little, a lot of people couldn't understand me, but now a lot of people could understand me. And the other girls, they wasn't teasing me so much anymore. How could they? Lots of them talked much worse.

I felt good when I knew my speech was getting better. It made me feel real good that people won't think maybe there's something wrong with me.

25

When I'm not in school, like in the afternoon, they let me out by myself. I could walk around the grounds, I could go to the canteen and listen to music. 'Cause I was older, 'cause I was going on grown-up, twenty years old now and gonna be twenty-one in winter. I wasn't getting into orneriness like I use to, I was behaving myself more than I use to.

If it's a nice day, I take a book and go set out on the front lawn under one of the trees and read. Or sometimes I have lots of fun looking for adventure, even go down by the hedge and watch the cars go by. It passes the time away and makes me wonder where all them cars are going to. Maybe to cities, maybe to countries, maybe to big farms.

One morning I'm setting in school. I was all done my arithmetic, so I was reading about Nancy Drew. The Nancy Drew books are hard sometimes and I do need help with words, but I like Nancy Drew. She gets into mystery. Ghosts and clocks and haunted houses, I love that stuff.

Mrs. Knopf come over to me, she set down in Gloria's seat and she said, "Put down your book, Winifred."

"But I'm all done my work. I'll show you."

"No, I wanna talk to you. I'm gonna start you in one of my special classes next week."

"What kind of special class?"

"Community Living. It teaches you about how to do things in the outside world. 'Cause maybe some day you'll be leaving the institution."

"And going back home?"

"I didn't say that, I don't know about that. Don't be getting all in a dither, Winifred." She was smiling at me. Mrs. Knopf has the kind of smile makes you feel she likes you. "You got to stay here for a long time, you got a lot of things to learn, still. I'm just talking about maybe."

So on regular days I go to school in the morning time like always, but on Wednesday afternoons, after I get my lunch, I go back for Community Living. We set at desks in the school room, me and some other girls. The only one I know is Shirley. And instead of doing spelling and arithmetic and geography, we start to learn about street signs.

Mrs. Knopf held up a big picture of a stop light with the green circle all lit up. "Who could tell what this is?" she asked us. We raise up our hands, we all call out, "Stop light!" That one was easy.

"What does it mean when the green is lit up? Don't call out, just raise up your hands."

She called on a girl and the girl said, "It means go," and then she held up a picture of a stop light, got the red all lit up, and we raised our hands again. She called on me.

"It means stop!" I said. I thought, hmmmm, this stuff is easy. But then she held up a picture of another stop light. This one got the middle lit up, the yellow part. No one raised hands.

"Don't anyone know what the yellow light means?"

We all just set there.

"Franny, do you know?"

"Nighttime?"

Mrs. Knopf said no, yellow light means the light is

changing from green to red, means you better stand still and wait, don't cross the street.

We learned about stop signs and railroad crossing signs. If you see RR XING, it means watch out or you could get run down by a train. We learned about danger signs and caution signs; they mean you better watch out, too. But not for trains.

Mrs. Knopf learned us about the calendar, which I mostly knew already, but still I set quiet and do my work. She told us the twelve months and what holidays they got, she told us the seasons and how many days in a week and how many weeks in a year. I forget how many now, but I know there's a lot. More than a hundred.

Then come telling time, and that did give me trouble. I could tell the hours and the half-hours, but the in-betweens is very difficult. Sometimes it's hard to count by fives, and that's how you have to do if someone says, "What time is it?" and it's twenty minutes past seven.

26

When Mrs. Knopf gets the orange and black paper from the supply closet, when Mrs. Knopf tells us to cut out pumpkins for the windows, that's how I know Halloween is coming.

Mrs. Knopf has a great big garden out back of her house and every year just before Halloween she brings in pumpkins, real pumpkins, that she growed just for us. She takes a knife and cuts them open real careful so the stem part comes off with the top, but the pumpkin don't get all messed up. Then we cover the desks with newspapers and she puts us into groups. We have to share the pumpkins. Mrs. Knopf don't have time to grow one for each girl. Last of all, she gives us big spoons so we could dig out the wet orange stuff and the seeds.

I tell Mrs. Knopf, "No spoon for me, thanks. I rather use my hands, just only my hands." I love to stick my hands down in that pumpkin, feel the cool, slippy insides. I love to get my hands full of that stuff and close my hands up tight so it squishes out my fingers. Sometimes I even stick my nose inside the pumpkin and go sniff, sniff, sniff. The other girls say, "What are you doing?" I say, "I'm smelling it!" They laugh to see me sniffing and sniffing, but it don't bother me none.

When we get the pumpkins all cleaned out we draw spooky faces on them, but my best part is cleaning them out. I don't care about doing the face.

Parties come at Halloween time, too. The outside ladies—the ones that come and do good things—they have parties for us sometimes on holidays.

Mrs. Treadwell told me and Shirley and Ruby Rose that we could go to the party in Meadow Building instead of going to the party in Children's Cottage. That's 'cause we was the oldest girls in Children's Cottage. Meadow is one of the grown-up buildings and that's where we're gonna get put when we finish up with school. Soon as you're out of school you can't stay in Children's Cottage no more.

We was thrilled to go to the party at Meadow 'cause they give you costumes to wear, real Halloween costumes. I never had a Halloween costume before, but I seen the grown-up girls wearing them. Some are real fine costumes. The girls in the Sewing Department, the girls who are learning to sew, they make them.

Mrs. Drake told us at supper time, "Tomorrow I'll take you kids over to the Sewing Department. We'll pick out some costumes for you."

* * *

Me and Ruby Rose couldn't go to sleep, we laid there in our beds talking about what we was gonna be. Ruby Rose said, "I'm gonna be a queen."

"Not me," I told her, "I'm gonna be Nancy Drew. Or a cat."

"Shut up so I could get my sleep," Dolly said.

I told Ruby Rose, "Oh, Dolly's jealous, Dolly wants a costume, too. Dolly wants to go to the grown-up party, but she can't. She's not old enough."

"You should wear a monkey costume," Dolly said, "'cause that's what you look like." She laughed, and some of the other kids laughed, too. Even Ruby Rose.

"Shut up," I told her, "stop laughing at me or I'll bop you."

Dolly kept laughing.

All the kids was setting up in bed. They know me, they know when a fight is coming. I jump out of bed, stomp over to Dolly's bed, grab her arm. Told her, "I'm gonna break your mouth off," and I start pulling her out of bed.

"You better not, you better not," she yowled, "or I won't let you see my book. I was gonna let you see my book, but now I'm not gonna let you see it!"

"What book?"

"The dirty book. That my brother give me."

"You don't have no dirty book!"

"Yes, I do. Ask Cora. Ask Bonnie."

Mrs. O'Brien come in then, got a bunch of socks in her hands. "What the heck is going on? What are you doing to Dolly?"

I let go Dolly's arm. "I can't help it, Mrs. O'Brien. She's jealous that we're getting costumes and I'm gonna bop her if she don't shut up about it."

"You get back in bed or Mrs. Treadwell's gonna hear about this tomorrow," she told me, "and Dolly, button your lip."

I got back into bed, but I give Dolly a real nasty look, and when Mrs. O'Brien bended over to pick up some socks she dropped I stuck out my tongue at her behind. Then I stuck out my tongue at Ruby Rose. She didn't have to go and laugh at me, too.

There wasn't a lot of costumes left, so we had to take what fit us. Shirley and Ruby Rose both had to be Mickey Mouse, got mouse suits that zipped and got Mickey Mouse masks with big round ears, the store kind. But I was lucky. I got the bunny rabbit costume 'cause I was the only one tall enough to fit it. It was gray, it zipped up, had hands and feets, too, and got them big, floppy bunny ears. Mrs. Drake showed me how to wear them, they got a string to tie under the chin. No mask, but I didn't care. I loved my costume. I thought it was gonna be such a thrill to be a bunny rabbit.

We kids got our supper early, then everyone went into the playroom to have their Halloween party. But not us.

I said to Dolly, "Bye-bye, it's time for me to put on my bunny rabbit costume."

Mrs. Drake helped us get dressed. First Shirley. She needed a lot of help 'cause she can't get out of her wheeling chair. Ruby Rose and me could dress ourselfs, but Mrs. Drake tied on my ears for me.

"You kids look great," she said. "Wanna see?" And she took us downstairs to the attendants' bathroom to look in the mirror. She was right, we did look great. Especially me. My face was the same, but the rest of me was bunny all over. I look in the mirror and went hop, hop, hop.

"Look at me, look at me," I said.

"Not fair," Shirley said, "I want to be a bunny too."

Ruby Rose just looked in the mirror, said, "I don't like mices."

"Hush, hush, let's go or you'll miss the food," Mrs. Drake said. That shut us up.

Mrs. Drake walked us over to Meadow and I pushed Shirley's wheeling chair. It was almost dark. It was exciting to be going someplace in the dark, going to a party, but the most exciting thing of all was to be going out looking like a bunny rabbit. Every now and then I give a little hop, then Shirley had to tell me to cut it out 'cause I wasn't pushing the wheeling chair straight.

"All Winifred needs now is a great big carrot," Mrs. Drake said. That made me laugh.

Oh boy, you should of seen them costumes. Cowboys and cowgirls and Superman and two tigers and some girls all dressed up in long gowns, got beads and jewelry and makeup, and one got a shiny crown on the head. There was a couple ghosts with sheets and a witch with a pointy hat and four more Mickey Mouses.

Mrs. Drake left us there in the Day Room at Meadow, time for her to go home. First we just set there looking at everyone. Seen a couple girls we knew, use to be in our building. Antonia got on some kind of costume, but we couldn't tell what it was. She was just setting in a corner with one of the tigers, looked like she didn't care if the world comes or goes. That's how Antonia is. Most of the others was talking and laughing, making jokes and pointing at each other and acting real silly. We just set there, you could say we was shy, and it was awful noisy.

The outside ladies was buzzing around; they all had pretty dresses, pretty hair. They was making a fuss over the girls, going up to everyone saying things like what a great costume, what a scary costume, isn't this a lot of fun? Then they started to dish out the goodies.

One of the Meadow attendants yelled for everyone to be quiet but you couldn't hardly hear her. So she banged and banged on one of the tables, yelled, "Quiet! I said QUIET!" Then everyone shut up.

"These ladies got ice cream and cake for you," she told us. "Anybody wants some, get in line. And remember to say 'thank you' to the nice ladies."

It was a long line. I was starting to feel hot inside my bunny costume, I thought we wasn't never gonna get to that food. When it come my turn, I give the lady my plate. She put a piece of cake on it, she said, "What kind of ice cream?" There was chocolate, vanilla and strawberry. I wished I could ask for all of it—a little chocolate, a little vanilla, a little strawberry—but I just said, "Chocolate," real polite, then I said, "Thank you."

We set at a little table. There was a couple others at the table, but they didn't pay us no mind, too busy eating. Ruby Rose and Shirley took off their masks and started to eat, too. But I couldn't eat. My hands was inside the bunny costume and I couldn't feed myself.

"I can't feed myself," I told Ruby Rose. She just kept eating her food. I set there and tried to think how to eat my ice cream and cake. I could eat like bunny rabbits eat.

I bit off a piece of my cake, but it fell out of my mouth, I didn't get much. My chocolate ice cream was starting to melt. Everyone else was busy gobbling up their food.

I took my plate over to one of the ladies, said, "Would you feed me? I can't feed myself." She had a friendly face, she had orange lipstick, she called me "sweetie." "Sweetie, can't you take off your costume?"

"But I don't have nothing underneath, no dress." I had to wear shoes, put my bunny rabbit feets inside my shoes, but I didn't have no dress on.

"Wait, I'll help you in a minute." She was putting cake and ice cream on some plates.

I was itching in my costume, I was hot and itchy. My ice cream was dripping off my plate and I didn't have no napkin. I was getting tired of being a bunny rabbit.

The lady took the plates to the corner where Antonia and the tiger was. She give them each a plate, got them spoons, then she come back. "Now I could feed you," she said. She fed me off my plate, my ice cream and cake, even give me a little more ice cream 'cause mine was so messy. Only this time I ask for strawberry.

I wanted to go home, back to my building, get off my costume. But then it come time for the contest. The attendant yelled "Quiet!" again, and she told everybody that now the ladies was gonna pick out the prettiest costume, the scariest costume and the funniest costume. And whoever was wearing them costumes, they would win a surprise.

The ones that wanted to be in the contest had to stand in line in the middle of the Day Room so the ladies could get a good look, so the ladies could make up their minds. The girls was laughing and dancing around, trying to show off, calling out, "Pick me! Pick me!" Some was acting real silly. One girl pulled up her gown to show the ladies her bloomers. But the ladies was real polite, acted like they didn't see. They just walked around, looked everybody over, then they set down at a table and whispered a little bit. When they was done whispering one of the ladies stood up, not the one with orange lipstick, and we was all quiet. We was waiting to know who was gonna win.

"First, I wanna tell you that you all got such beautiful costumes, you all look so good," she said.

The girls clapped, the girls cheered, some of the girls whistled. The attendant yelled, "QUIET!"

"The winner of the scariest costume is the witch!"

The girl in the witch costume clapped real hard when the lady said that, but nobody else did. The lady give her a little present wrapped in white paper and she opened it and it was a box of colored pencils.

"Next comes the winner of the funniest costume," the lady said. "It's the bunny rabbit!" I looked all around at the other girls, then I remember the bunny rabbit is me. I won!

"I'm the bunny rabbit, I'm the bunny rabbit!" and I go hop, hop, hop. The lady laughed when she give me my present. "I won, I won," I kept yelling, almost forgot to open my present. It was in pretty white paper like the pencils, but it wasn't pencils, it was a pink comb. I really liked it. I showed it to Ruby Rose, I showed it to Shirley, they said it was a nice comb. I didn't hear who won the last surprise, didn't even care. I was just so proud.

★ ★ ★

The outside ladies said bye-bye to everyone. Said they'd come back soon, and they left. But still the party wasn't over. One of the attendants plugged in the Victrola and the girls start putting on records, dancing with each other. Antonia was still setting in the corner, she was all by herself, looked to me to be asleep. Or thinking with her eyes closed.

The music made an awful racket and I was tired and hot and itchy. I was glad when Mrs. O'Brien come to take us back to Children's Cottage.

I laid there in bed, just couldn't get to sleep. Seemed like nobody was awake but me. I set up and looked over at Dolly. She was real still. I watched her for a little bit. It sure seemed like she was sleeping.

I got out of bed real slow and tippytoed over to Dolly's bed. It was quiet. No one talking in their sleep, no one having bad dreams. Dolly was laying there with her eyes closed, she was all covered up and making little snorings. I set down on the floor and pulled the Belongings Box out from under her bed, took everything out of it real fast. I was scared someone might come in.

She got some old candy in there, got a birthday card, a couple pieces of puzzle, a whole bunch of sticks and some comics. And a fat little book that was under the comics. I sticked the fat little book in my nightie, then I put everything back fast as I could.

The light was on in the Clothing Room. I could hear Mrs. Samuels and Mrs. O'Brien in there, must be they was laying out our stuff for morning.

Couldn't go in the bathroom, no privacy there.

I tippytoed down the hall, got the book still under my nightie, holding it close to my tummy so it couldn't fall. I went into the cleaning closet, pulled the string to make the light come on, closed the door.

It wasn't a real book, it was more like comics. Cartoon pictures. Only they wasn't animals or kids or funny things, they was ladies and men. And was they ever doing dirty things to each other. I'm no dummy, I know the birds and the bees. The grown-up girls talk about that stuff all the time, make up stories about the boys from Kortland that they dance with. But some of them pictures got people doing things I never heard of, shameful terrible things. The book had words, too, in them kind of balloons that come from people's heads, and most of the words I could read.

I'm setting on the floor in the closet, turning pages, so busy I forget where I am. Bam, the door opens, and there's Mrs. O'Brien. She stood there a minute looking at me, then she said, "Give me that book."

"I don't have to."

"Winifred, you give me that book."

"No, I won't. 'Cause it isn't mine."

She leaned down like to grab it, so I threw it in the corner behind the buckets. She cussed me, she pulled me up by the hair.

"Leave go my hair!" I scream, and I called her something bad. I can't say what it was, but it was one of the words that was in the book.

She grabbed the dustbroom off the shelf and started to hit me, hitting me and beating me with the dustbroom. Right on the breast, too. I give her a push, run out of the closet. Some of the kids was there, must of woke up from the yelling and come to see. I run down to the Clothing Room screaming, "Mrs. Samuels! Mrs. Samuels!" But no one was there. Then I seen her running up the stairs.

"What happened, Winifred?"

But I couldn't tell her. I was too upset, in hysterical crying. She sent one of the kids down to get Mrs. Weissman, the night supervisor, then she took me to my bed, made me set down. When Mrs. Weissman come she ask me what happened, too, but I could hardly talk for crying. One of the kids, Annie, told that Mrs. O'Brien beat me up with a dustbroom.

"A what?"

"This," Ruby Rose said, and she give Mrs. Weissman the dustbroom. It was broke in two pieces.

"She put it on the top shelf to hide it," Annie said. "But we found it."

In the morning time I didn't have to get up, they let me stay in bed. I had a big black and blue on my breast and they kept putting ice packs on it so I wouldn't get cancer. Also had to give me pills for my nerves.

Mrs. Drake and Miss Emmett was so nice to me, brung me special cookies and juice in bed, set and talked to me. I heard Mrs. Drake tell Miss Emmett no wonder Winifred's so nervous, getting beat up with a dustbroom. And she's only a young kid just got out of her teen age.

Mrs. Treadwell come to see me. She wasn't well, had some kind of dropsies in her feets and they was all swollen. She set on my bed, asked me what I done to get Mrs. O'Brien so mad. I told her the truth, too, told her I was looking at a dirty book in the closet and wouldn't give it to her.

"Who give you the book, Winifred?"

"I found it." I don't think that was really a lie, I did find it. She looked like she was gonna ask me something else about finding it, so I said real quick, "Mrs. Treadwell, I'm sorry about all the screaming I done, but I couldn't help it. It was mercy screaming."

"You sure do scream loud," she said. "They heard you clear over to Grove Building."

"I bet no one else screams like that."

"Get some rest, Winifred," she told me.

They fired Mrs. O'Brien, boy, she got fired. They said they don't allow people who bang people around. I don't know what happened to Dolly's book, but I bet she never got it back.

27

I thought I was dreaming when I read the letter Gladys sent me. She said she was coming to get me, take me to her house for Thanksgiving so I could meet her husband, meet her babies. That was the best letter I ever got.

The attendants packed me. I was all ready when Gladys come.

"Oh, you're ready," Gladys said.

"What do you mean, ready?" I told her. "I been ready all day."

Gladys looked so good to me, she did. Pretty in the face, nice red hair. She was getting a little on the plump side. She put my bag in the back seat.

"Where's your husband? Where's your babies?"

"Clayton's working, Winnie," she said. "You'll meet him tonight. And I left the kids home 'cause this trip is too long for them."

Off we go in the car. It was so good to get away from the institution, so good to be out in the world again. I love riding in a car, I do. Wish I could ride in a car every single day.

Gladys's house was nice, it was small and white. I told her, "Oh, Gladys, you got a nice house."

The inside was nice, too. Not as pretty as the McKennas', but I didn't tell Gladys that. She got a couple little rugs, but not in every room, and got a little kitchen, a little dining room, a little living room with a television in it, and a little upstairs. I liked it that she had a television. We got one at the institution now, in the playroom, and I sure do enjoy watching it.

Her babies was in the kitchen. A girl, a girl that was taking care of them, was giving them their supper. "Winnie, this here's Hannah and this here's Marina," Gladys told me. And looked at them babies like she really did love them. They was glad to see her, too. They was pretty kids, and the little one got the same red hair Gladys got.

She told the kids, "This here's your Aunt Winnie." I said, "Who?" and she said, "Winnie, you're their aunt." I was surprised. I didn't think I could be no one's aunt. Gladys said I had to be their aunt 'cause I was the sister of their mother. I said okay, that was okay by me. I liked the idea.

After the girl left, Gladys put the kids to bed. Hannah had to show me how she could put her own stuff on, said, "No, no, no," if you tried to help. But I helped put the diapers on Marina, and the nightie.

Gladys didn't know I could diaper, said, "How did you learn to do that?" I was real proud, I told her, "Well, sometimes I help diaper my friend Jeannie, so that's how I learned to do it!"

Gladys made us some supper, hamburgers and baked beans. I could see in the ice box she had all the yummy stuff for Thanksgiving, such as turkey and pies.

"Could I look at television?" I ask her, and she said, "Sure. We could even eat our supper by the television if you want." And she fixed us up a little table right in front of the television set and she turned off all the lights in the living room. We ate our hamburgers and baked beans, doughnuts for dessert, and watched a show where people answer questions the man asks and if they give him the right answer, he gives them a whole bunch of money. They was hard questions, but some of the people could answer all of them. Real smart people.

It was such a treat for me to eat my supper and look at television programs at the same time. Gladys said she done that whenever Clayton was away, eat with the television. I told her, "Oh, Gladys, you're lucky."

Clayton come home late from his truck. I was setting in

the chair by the television and I was almost asleep, it was past my bedtime. I was happy to meet him, but he didn't say much. He looked real tired, too.

I slept in a cot next to the crib in the babies' room. It was a hard cot but I didn't mind, and Gladys let me have two pillows. Marina kept making little baby sounds. A couple times she cried and I had to get up, find the bottle for her, 'cause it would drop on the floor. Then she'd start in sucking real loud until she fell back to sleep.

Next morning Gladys said to me, "Winnie, Miriam and Willy is coming today and guess who else."

"Who else?"

"The Krullers."

"The Krullers? My mother and daddy?"

"Yes," Gladys said. "I didn't want to tell you last night, I was afraid you was gonna be so excited and nervous you wouldn't get no sleep."

She was right, I did get excited and nervous. I didn't see my mother and daddy for years and years. I thought I wasn't never gonna see them again.

I helped with the cooking, I helped with the babies, but all the day I kept thinking about that I was gonna see my mother and daddy. Couldn't keep my mind on nothing else. I tripped over a chair, I dropped the forks, I spilled Hannah's milk. Clayton give me a look, he thought I was clumsy. Lunchtime come, I couldn't even eat all my food.

Miriam and Willy come first. I was real happy to see Miriam. I didn't see her since I was little, but she did write to me a couple times. I told her, "Miriam, I didn't see you in so long I forgot what you look like!" She said she forgot what I look like, too.

She introduced me to her husband, we shake hands, and he smile like he's a real polite man. Then Hannah run to her and Miriam had to pick her up. Hannah kept singing, "Hi,

Aunt Miriam, hi, Aunt Miriam." Hannah called Miriam "aunt" too, must be 'cause she's another sister of Gladys's.

We all set in the living room and ate peanuts and pretzels. Clayton brung out beer and soda for everyone and I had soda. We was all talking. Miriam was asking me questions about how was I, and I was telling her, but all I could think of was my mother and daddy, that I was going to see them.

Then we heard a car out front and Gladys said, "Here they are!"

Clayton went to open the door for them and then everyone was yelling "hello" and "Happy Thanksgiving" and my mother said, "I could smell that turkey cooking all the way outside!" I run to my daddy, I didn't go to my mother. He put his arms around me, hugged me tight. He looked the same to me, he looked just like always, and so did my mother. He said, "Winnie, it's good to see you."

My mother said, "My God, how fast kids grow."

"I'm not a kid no more," I told her. "I'm almost twenty-one."

"Twenty-one," my daddy said. "Last time we seen you was when we come down in the summer, you was about thirteen or fourteen."

"Seven years," my mother said.

Clayton took their coats upstairs and we all set down again. Gladys got some more stuff for everyone to eat and drink. My mother tried to get Hannah to set on her lap, but she wouldn't. She was shy of her.

"Are they treating you okay there?" my mother asked me.

"Not too good."

"You're so skinny," she said.

"I don't get enough to eat."

They all talked about the babies and about what Wanda was doing, and then Miriam and Gladys went into the kitchen to get dinner ready. Marina woke up from her nap and started hollering, so I went up to get her, and she did set in my mother's lap. My mother made a big fuss about her. Saying things like isn't she sweet, isn't she pretty, look at all that red hair.

I was getting mad watching my mother be so nice to Marina. I thought, well, maybe she don't want to bother with me 'cause she's not my real mother. Big deal. I don't give a darn if she's my foster mother. Let her be my foster mother, she could take my real mother's place, couldn't she? Somebody has to be my mother.

I said to her real loud, "It'll be another seven years before I see you again."

Everybody looked at me, then they started to laugh. Thought I was being funny. My mother said, "No, it won't be."

"Oh, yes it will."

That's the last time I seen her and it's a lot more than seven years now.

I was a big help to Gladys after everybody left. Helped her do the dishes, put away the food, clean up the whole kitchen. It was raining out, raining hard. Clayton and the babies was upstairs asleep.

"You don't want me," I told Gladys. "That's why I'm in the institution. Maybe you think I'm mentally retarded or something."

"Is that why you're looking so blue?" Gladys got clean towels and we start drying up the pots. "So what if you're in an institution, I still love you. And you're not gonna be there all your life. You'll get a chance to be out."

"When?"

"I don't know, Winnie."

After we got the pots all dried out she made us some Lipton tea and we set down at the kitchen table. She took off her shoes. "Sure is good to set," she said.

I put lots of sugar in my tea. I like lots of sugar.

"You wasn't doing much talking," Gladys said. "Did you like the dinner?"

"If my parents was alive, I bet I wouldn't be put in no

institution," I told her. "If my parents was alive, I bet I would be home."

"Maybe so, Winnie."

"Why did they have to die on me?"

I thought Gladys wasn't gonna tell me nothing. She drunk some of her tea, but then she said, "Well, mama was sick a long time. She died when you was two. In the spring daddy got pneumonia and he died."

"Who took care of us when daddy died?"

"Gram come to live with us for a little while, Gram Olesky. But she was too old to do all that work, so we went to the Krullers'."

"I remember her, I remember Gram. Why didn't she never come see me in the institution?"

"I think the trip was just too much for her."

I couldn't go to sleep. The windows was shaking from the wind and rain and it was cold in the house even under the covers. Couldn't get my feets to feeling warm. Then Marina started to cry, dropped her bottle again. I got out of the cot, even with my cold feets, got the bottle and give it back to her. I didn't mind, I was glad to be an aunt.

28

Mrs. Knopf put the folders in a big thing like an envelope, Mrs. Knopf told me to ask for Miss Marise when I got to the Office Building, give the folders to her.

"Remember. Miss Marise."

"Don't worry, I'll remember."

I walked slow. It was a good-feeling day. Sunny and warm, not like winter was almost coming. Didn't hardly need a coat. I carried the envelope real careful, I made sure it didn't drop. Doing an errand is an important thing. I could tell Mrs. Knopf trusted me to do a good job.

When I got to the Office Building, I done just like Mrs. Knopf said to do. "I wanna see Miss Marise, please," I told the lady at the front desk. She took me into a little office where there was another lady.

"I wanna see Miss Marise, please," I said.

"I'm Miss Marise."

"Well, this here's for you. Mrs. Knopf told me to bring it to you."

I put the big envelope on her desk. She said, "Thank you." I told her, "Oh, that's okay, that's okay."

I walk back to school by the longest way. Kicked up piles of leafs and laughed to see them go flying in the air. The low-grades was out sunning theirselfs at Forest and Mrs. Paretti was setting on a bench in the yard sewing. I went over to the fence, called, "Hi, Mrs. Paretti."

"Oh, Winifred, hi."

"How's Jeannie?"

"Go see her, she's right over there." I went into the yard. "Haven't seen you in a long time, Winifred."

"I been real busy. School and Community Living. Went away to visit my sister, too."

There was some wheeling chairs setting by the building and Jeannie was in one of them. "Hi, Jeannie," I said. Jeannie looked at me, then she waved her hands and laughed. When she laughed like that, she slobbered. "It's me, it's Winifred," I said. Jeannie just kept waving her hands around. I went back and set down next to Mrs. Paretti.

"I just run an errand for Mrs. Knopf," I told her.

"Oh, you're running errands now?"

"I sure am."

"How's school?"

"Good. I'm doing good. And I go to Community Living on Wednesdays, too."

"What are they teaching you?"

"About money now. You know, nickels, quarters, dimes. We gotta learn which is which."

"Oh, that's real nice."

"Well, I gotta go back to school now, Mrs. Paretti. I think Mrs. Knopf is waiting on me."

I yelled, "Bye, Jeannie!" Jeannie was still waving.

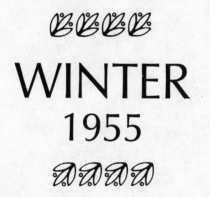

WINTER
1955

29

I wish I had a real mother and father, 'cause I need one. Seems like everyone has a real mother but me. Sometimes I like to set and think about my mother. I think, what was she like? Was she pretty?

If I had a mother, I'd let you know, boy. I wouldn't be out of her sight not one day, I'd be always about her, on her apron strings. I would stay with her until the day she pass away. My greatest wish is mother love, I'd give all the money in the world for mother love.

I told Dr. Kravitz—he's my psychiatrist now, I go to him every Friday in the Psychology Department—I told Dr. Kravitz I think my life would be much more different from what it is if my real mother was alive. Maybe I wouldn't be the black sheep of the family, the nervous type. Maybe I wouldn't get upset so easy, carry on and do bad things like I done when I was little. Hitting kids. I told Dr. Kravitz sometimes kids aren't bad when they get love.

I wish I was a normal kid. Normal kids are nice and there's nothing wrong with them. But nobody's perfect, I guess.

Only thing I don't like about living in Meadow is roll call. Roll call is a check to see if we're all here. And I hate it. Everybody has to stand by their bed and when the attendant calls out your name you gotta say "Here." Then she checks you off her list. Every darn time you turn around they're doing roll call. At night, in the morning, when you come back from the cafeteria or Assembly Hall, always checking to see if we're in or we're not in. Makes me feel like I'm in jail.

I liked the other things about Meadow, liked it that it was a real grown-up building. It made me feel grown-up. And it's fun to go to the cafeteria to get your food instead of just eating in the basement like you do in Children's Cottage. The cafeteria is big, it's noisy, but I like to get my tray, I like to stand in line. Then the people behind the counter gives you all your food, you get your fork and spoon, you go set with your friends to eat. It puts me in mind of a restaurant, a real restaurant. And at Christmastime, they hang red and green paper from the ceiling and got a big picture of Santa Claus on the door where you come in.

Me and Ruby Rose was walking back to Meadow after lunch, Kissy was with us too. She got her baby doll stuck down inside her coat, keep it from the wind.

"Kissy's going home," she told us. "My mommy is coming, take Kissy home." Kissy is grandmother age, fifty or seventy years old, wrinkles on the face and white hair. She's one of them real peculiar ones. Her name is Christina, I know that from roll call, but she don't know it. She's not too smart, or could be she can't say it right, has to call herself Kissy.

"Your mommy isn't coming," I told her. "You don't even have a mommy. You're too old."

"Yes, yes, Kissy's going home," she said.

"She thinks she's going home," I told Ruby Rose. Lots of girls do that, keep telling you they're going home tomorrow, but tomorrow comes and they will still be there. They're not going nowhere. After awhile you know not to believe them no more, but that don't stop them. They keep right on telling you.

"She is going home," Ruby Rose said.

"No, she isn't, that's just how she's always saying."

"Yes, she is. Some of her family is coming after her for Christmas. Mrs. Potts said."

We put our coats away and me and Ruby Rose went into the Day Room. Some of the girls was watching a soap opera on television. Kissy come in with her coat still on, didn't have the brains to take it off. She set down on the couch near to us, rocked her baby doll.

"Everybody's going home for Christmas," I said.

"No, they're not."

"It's no fair," I said, "even Kissy's going home for Christmas."

Ruby Rose set there looking at the television, said, "I wish I could go home too, but I don't hear from my mother no more. Maybe she went to Philadelphia."

I didn't feel like watching television, anyway I think them soap operas is trash. I went upstairs to get my book. I don't go to school no more, but Mrs. Knopf still lets me take books from the library. She knows I'm real careful and always bring them back in time. I was reading about the Bobbsey Twins. Boy, I love them books, I must of read five or six of them Bobbsey Twins books.

I brung the book down to the Day Room, but I was just feeling too blue to read. My family never once took me home for Christmas, only Mrs. McKenna a long, long time ago. Every Christmas here I am, stuck in this darn institution.

I wished I could just run away.

30

When Mrs. Potts told me I was on the list for the dance this month, I told her I didn't even want to go. Told her I can't dance, and anyway I would be too shy. She said, "Give it a try, Winifred."

All the girls was dressed up pretty. Some even had lipstick on. I guess they was allowed to do that for special. Franny got on a real pretty dress and her hair curled up. She wanted to get me fixed up too, curl my hair, take off my glasses. I told her, "I don't want my hair curled. God made me look this way and I have to take what God give me. Anyway, I know no one's gonna think I'm pretty."

I put my hair up in a ponytail, though, and I washed my face real good.

In the Assembly Hall they got tables and chairs set up by the stage, the rest of the place was clear for dancing. We set around waiting for the boys to come. I was nervous, I was scared maybe some boy would try to talk to me. You could say I wasn't use to boys, wasn't use to talking to them. Maybe they would make fun of me. I heard boys might do that to people.

The other girls was all in a dither. Billie was talking real loud about that her sweetheart was saving all his money to get her a ring for Christmas. Showing off. She's got a sweetheart name Aldo she's always talking and boasting about. Aldo, Aldo, Aldo, that's all you ever hear from her. Some of the girls was telling dirty jokes about the boys, laughing real hard, and some was setting there worrying did their dress look right, did their hair look pretty or not. I just bit my nails.

Someone yelled, "The bus! The bus!" Everyone jump up, run to the door, knocked over a couple chairs getting there. I went, too, 'cause I didn't wanna stay alone at the table.

Outside it was starting to snow a little, and there was the brown bus, said KORTLAND on it. The boys was getting off and lining up with their attendants, then they come marching into the Assembly Hall, waving and shouting to the girls. The girls was clapping and jumping up and down, some was looking for their sweethearts. So much fuss, so much pushing and jumping, I thought I was gonna get hurt. I was getting a sick headache.

When the boys was all inside the attendants hollered, "Shut up and set down!" It took awhile, but everyone did shut up and set down after the attendants said they wasn't gonna start the music until it was quiet.

They started playing records and I just stood there, watched the people dancing. You should of seen Billie and Aldo, they was dancing like they was sticked together. Aldo was short, fat too, didn't look to me like nothing to boast about. Some of the girls who didn't have no partners was dancing together, so was some of the boys. Then come the fast music and everyone was hopping all around together. I didn't know what the heck to do with myself, only just wanted to go back to my building. I was glad when they turned the Victrola off, I was glad when one of the attendants hollered, "Snack time!" Everybody run back to the tables in a hurry.

I set with Franny and Lucy and some other girls who didn't have sweethearts. Some boys from Kortland was at our table, too. One of them set right next to me. The attendants was going around to all the tables giving everyone a paper plate with a cupcake and some apple slices, also passed out orange juice. For awhile it was real quiet. Everyone was busy eating their food.

The boy next to me said, "It's snowing outside."

I kept eating my cupcake. And all the while I was eating, that boy was looking at me. I tried to keep my face down. Franny said, "Oooh, I think he likes you." I told her, "Shut up, Franny."

When we was all done our food, juice too, the boy ask me, "What's your name?"

"Winifred."

"Well, Winifred, we had ham for dinner tonight. What did you have?"

"Spanish rice."

"Sunday we had applesauce." He was smiling all the while he was talking to me. He looked old, gray hair, nice smiley blue eyes with glasses, and a kind face. Polite, too.

It was getting noisy again, people starting to talk and laugh and run around. Some boys was ganged up chasing girls around the tables. I seen one girl kick a boy when he catched her. Kicked him right in the privates. The boy set down on the floor and cried, then an attendant had to come and help him get up, took him away. That boy looked like he was really hurting.

"Are you shy?"

"Nope," I said, "I'm not shy."

"Well, sometimes I'm shy of girls, but I'm not shy of you." Then they turned the Victrola on again, a cowboy song, and he said, "Would you dance with me?"

"No. I can't dance." Franny and Lucy kept telling me, "Go on, go on." I was wishing they'd shut up their darn mouths.

"Come on." He pull me right out of my chair. I said, "No, no," but I was laughing, couldn't help myself. "See, dancing's easy," he said, but I just kept laughing. Tried to move my feets like he was moving his feets, but it wasn't easy, and he had his arms around me and that was hard to get use to. It made me feel real silly, it did, that he had his arms around me. He said, "Do you like me? I like you." But I couldn't answer for laughing.

When the song was done, we went back to the table and the boy pulled my chair out, make it more easy for me to set on it. Franny and Lucy wasn't there. I was glad.

"You know, Winifred, I'm real happy I met you."

"You are?"

"I'm lonely, I don't hardly have no family."

"You don't?"

"Only got a sister in Arizona, but she don't bother with me."

"Oh, I got a sister, too."

"No one writes to me," he said. "Would you write to me?"

"Okay." It was coming easy, the talking part. I was thinking of things to say.

He got a pen from one of the attendants, wrote down his address, name of his building on a napkin, then I wrote down my address, name of my building, on another napkin. I read his napkin. It said his name was Thomas Karr.

I told him, "You got a nice name."

"I'm sixty-one years old."

"That's okay."

"Would you dance with me next time we have a dance?"

"Sure I will."

When it come time for the boys to go, I went to the coat racks with him, help him find his coat. He held my hand. There was funny noises coming from behind the coats. We peep around and seen a boy and a girl back there. The boy was tickling the girl all over. Under the arms and every-place. And they was laughing. I know that girl, too, she's from Spruce Building.

Thomas put his coat on. He told me, "Winifred, you got a nice face."

"I do? I do have a nice face?"

"Would you be my girl?"

I told him, "Sure, Thomas. Any day!"

Some of the girls was getting letters from their families, or phone calls, telling them they was coming home for Christmas. I wrote to Gladys, ask could I please come to her for Christmas? Next week she wrote back, said I couldn't come 'cause they was going to Baltimore, have Christmas there with Clayton's family. Said she's gonna come see me on Saturday, though, and take me shopping for my Christmas present.

We went to Sears. I love Sears, you could buy anything there. It's a little like Woolworth's. Anything you could think of, I bet, they got in that store.

Gladys ask me what kind of present did I want for Christmas. I told her clothes, I want some pretty clothes. So we went to where all the clothes was and I picked out a beautiful blouse, white with a red ribbon on it, and got a black skirt to go with it. I tried the stuff on behind one of them little curtains, make sure it was fitting me right. Gladys said, "Winnie, you look real good in them clothes." I said, "Thank you!"

Then she took me to the diner for a little snack, yummy pie and tea. She showed me pictures of her kids, her little girls, and I told her I got a sweetheart now. She ask me all about Thomas, she teased me, made big eyes at me, said, "Oh, Winnie's in love!" I told her, "Stop it, stop laughing, Gladys!" but I was laughing too. I was so happy to be with Gladys. I do love Gladys.

When she was driving me back to the institution, I ask her, "How come you visit me and take me places and nobody else visits me and takes me places?"

"Well, Miriam's busy a lot, and Wanda lives far away."

"I don't think they like me. I think you're the only one likes me."

"They like you, Winnie. I just like you best. You was always special to me."

"I was special to you? Why was I special to you?"

"'Cause I'm the one took care of you when you was little. When mama was sick."

"Did you feed me?"

"Fed you, dressed you, even after Gram come I took care of you. When you got measles I put you in a wagon and took you to a doctor. Gram wouldn't go near you. She was scared she'd get measles."

"Did you take care of Miriam and Wanda, too?"

"Not as much as you. You was sickly a lot 'cause you was born too soon."

I give Gladys a big kiss when we got back to Meadow, told her, "Thanks for the pretty clothes, thanks for taking care of me when I was a baby."

She kissed me too, said, "Merry Christmas, Winnie, and you tell Thomas your sister Gladys says hello!"

★   ★   ★

I got a card from Miriam for Christmas and she sent me five dollars. That sure was nice of her. She never done that before.

Letter come from Thomas, too, he didn't even give me the chance to write first. He had nice handwriting. He wrote me about his job at Kortland, every morning he works in the hospital there mopping up the floors. He wrote that he has a little money—the institution pays him some for his work—and he was gonna buy me something when he got enough money saved up. Also he sent me a picture of him. But it wasn't a good picture, or could be it come from a long time ago, 'cause he looked real young.

I wrote right back. Told him about my job and also I'm working for Mrs. Knopf three times a week. Told him I had a real fine time at the dance. I said thank you for the picture, said I sure liked it, but I couldn't send him a picture of me 'cause I didn't have none.

I sticked his picture up over my bed with Scotch tape like Billie done with Aldo's picture. The girls right away start teasing me, not fun teasing like Gladys done, it was nasty teasing. Saying me and Thomas do bad things together. Talking dirty about us. That made me sick, it did, and if Mrs. Gaynor wasn't there I think I would of smacked about three of them in the head.

Anyway, Billie and Amelia got no rights to be teasing me about dirty things. I know what they do together in the nighttimes. Everyone knows.

31

They was dogging me to death when I got up, telling me I yelled out in my sleep all night, telling me I kept everyone awake.

"Can't you shut up even in the night?" Billie said.

"I can't help it," I told her. "When you're asleep you don't know what you're doing in your sleep, do you?"

Edith said, "Well, next time I'm gonna wake you up."

"You better not wake me up," I told her in a growly way. "That makes people very annoying."

I didn't even know what the heck I was yelling out. I guess whatever is on my mind in the daytime I yell out at night. And many a times I have nightmares, bad dreams about animals such as bears and tigers. Chasing me. Sometimes the curtain scares me, the curtain down the end of the dorm looks like a man standing there. Then I get nightmares about something is behind that curtain, something scary. Maybe when I have them bad dreams that makes me call out in my sleep. Is that my fault?

I got my soap, got my towel, went to wait for one of the showers to be empty. You got your choice, tub or shower. I like showers best, even if I have to wait longer. I like to stand there with the water coming down all over me. It feels like I'm outside in the rain.

When I come out I dried myself off, I put my towel around me, went back to the dorm to get my clothes. The girls was all getting dressed and they started in on me again, all of them talking about how nobody can't sleep 'cause of Winifred. They love to go after me. They know my nerves is bad, they know I'm gonna get real mad.

I told them, "I'm not the only one makes noises at night, other girls make noises, some girls get the fits! Why pick on me?"

"'Cause you're the only one that's a skinny-minny," Billie said.

I hit her, I bopped her one, and when I done that my towel dropped. All the girls that was in there—Billie, Amelia, Rita, Lucy, Edith—they laughed and clapped and whistled. I pulled up my towel, I bopped Billie again. I was crying.

Mrs. Gaynor and Mrs. Potts come in, made me stop. They told me to get dressed—I was shivering—then Mrs.

Gaynor took me and Billie down to Mrs. Demerest. Mrs. Demerest give us a talking to. She told me I gotta learn to stop smacking people and girls when I'm mad, I gotta get control over my tampers. She told me to stop crying and go wash my face with cold water.

I said, "I can't help it, Mrs. Demerest. How would you feel always stuck in this place even at Christmas? I'm sick of this place and I'm sick of living with a bunch of nasty girls!"

"That's enough, Winifred," she said, "calm down."

Then she told Billie she better not be picking on me no more, she told Billie, "When a girl's asleep she can't help what she's saying. So you just leave Winifred alone. How would you like to live in my house, 'cause we got a maid who walks in her sleep and she sings."

Dr. Kravitz is the best psychiatrist. He can read people's minds and he's mostly for disturbed girls and the nervous types, too. I know 'cause I'm the nervous type.

I told Dr. Kravitz the girls was bothering me something terrible, told him, "I'm sick of this institution. I'm sick of all them nasty girls and all them rules and all them attendants always bossing you."

He give me a cigarette. I learned to smoke from the big girls when I was fourteen, but I don't smoke much. Mostly, I just smoke in Dr. Kravitz's office 'cause he gives me cigarettes. He smokes a lot, he smokes too much, but he's handsome.

When I first started going to Dr. Kravitz I wouldn't tell him nothing, set there in that big chair with my mouth stuck shut. I couldn't trust him, he was just a new man to me. So he done all the talking. Told me I have to try and trust him, have faith in him. Told me he's helped other girls like me and he knows all about helping out my problems. He talked to me soft and kind and give me plenty of cigarettes.

But it's so hard to tell if you could trust people. One way to tell if you could trust someone is if you talk to them about someone else, then you have to wait a couple days to see if it gets back to the person you was talking about. Also, people you could trust, they set and talk with you, they hold conversation with you, they agree with you. Or sometimes you just look at someone and you say, yes, there's someone I could trust. It's this feeling you have, it's the way their eyes look at you. Dr. Kravitz has trustworthy eyes. So that's how I figured out I could trust him.

"Is that why you're looking so gloomy today?" he ask me. "'Cause you're sick of the institution?"

"I sure am, Dr. Kravitz. I wanna be in the outside world with people that's like normal people. Do exciting things like they do, go different places. Have pajama parties."

"Well, maybe when you learn to get along a little better, maybe when you get some more training, you could do them things."

"I'm tired of waiting! It's coming near Christmastime. Would you want to be in an institution at Christmastime?"

He said, "No."

We was all in our nighties lined up by our beds. Mrs. Gaynor was down the other end of the dorm doing roll call, and when she come to my name I didn't answer. I was feeling too fed up to do roll call.

She called again, "Winifred Sprockett! Where's Winifred? I thought I seen her up here."

Still I wasn't saying nothing.

"She's here," Ruby Rose said.

Mrs. Gaynor seen me, said, "Winifred, is your hearing gone bad? You got potatoes in your ears or something?"

"I could hear you."

"So why aren't you answering?"

"'Cause I'm tired of saying 'here,' 'here,' 'here,' all the time," I told her. "Don't you ever get tired of saying 'hello' to all the girls? Well, the girls is getting tired of saying 'here'!"

The girls started cheering me, they start hollering, "Yea,

Winifred!" Even Billie. And that really did surprise me. Didn't help me none, though. First thing in the morning back down to Mrs. Demerest I go, and this time I get punished. Stay in all day and scrub the bathroom floors.

I told Ruby Rose, "I'm running away. I had it with this place. I'm getting out of here."

"You'll get in trouble," she said.

"Only if they catch me. But they aren't gonna catch me."

"Where you gonna run to?"

"I don't know yet. I gotta think about it, make my plan."

I thought about it for days. When I was working, when I was eating, when I was laying in my bed. Hmmmm, couldn't go to Gladys's house, they wasn't gonna be home. Couldn't go to Miriam's house, she would send me right back to the institution. I'm not special to Miriam like I'm special to Gladys. Mrs. McKenna likes me, but she wouldn't let me stay, neither. She would know I was doing wrong.

And that's all the people I know on the outside. So I would have to go someplace where I didn't know no one. I could get me a job. The institution give me training in cleaning, a little sewing. And Mrs. Knopf learned me how to take phone messages. I could even wash dishes in a restaurant, maybe. I know girls who run away. Some get catched, but some don't. They never come back, they stay out in freedom. Oh, I wanted to be out in freedom, too!

Only thing, I would have to live all alone by myself. I wouldn't like living by myself. It's loneliness. And I would be so scared I would have to lock all the doors and windows.

I told Ruby Rose, "You should come with me."

"I don't want to."

"But maybe we could find your mother."

"Where?"

"In Philadelphia."

"How do you know she's in Philadelphia?"

"'Cause you told me that, dummy, don't you remember?"

"I did?"

I had some money saved up. Five dollars from what Miriam sent me and four dollars from what the institution give me each month for working. Five dollars and four dollars is nine dollars.

I ask Ruby Rose, "How much you got?" Ruby Rose is a sweeper, she gets paid for sweeping the building.

"I don't know. I gotta ask Mrs. Demerest to look it up."

"Go ask her, then."

Ruby Rose come back to the Day Room, said, "Four dollars. She says I got four dollars."

Nine dollars and four dollars is thirteen dollars. I told her, "We got thirteen dollars. That's enough to run away with."

"But I told you. I don't want to run away."

"Do you wanna find your mother?"

"Yes."

"Do you wanna have pajama parties? And go to the movies?"

"Oh, yes!"

"Then you better come with me."

First it was rainy, then it was snowy, then it come rainy some more. So we had to wait 'cause we didn't want to be out in bad weather. We didn't have no raincoats or umbrellas, no boots.

Then, no more rain, no more snow. I told Ruby Rose, "Bring your money when we go to the cafeteria 'cause we're gonna run away after supper."

Running away was easy as pies. Got our supper with all the other girls, then when we was done we just walk right off the grounds. Didn't take nothing with us but our money and ourselfs, didn't have nothing much to take, anyway. I was wearing my new clothes from Gladys, but most of our clothes is the institution's.

It was dark already, it was cold. Not much cars out. We

walked and walked up the road, then Ruby Rose set down and wouldn't go no more. Said, "I gotta stop walking, it's hurting." Most of the times she gets around real good, you forget there's a brace on her leg. But sometimes she don't get around real good. I told her, "Okay. Now I'm gonna stick up my thumb." I know that's how you make cars stop. I seen it on television.

First thing, we had to wait for a car to come. Then I sticked up my thumb. But it didn't make the car stop. Next time I seen car lights coming I jump right out into the road, make sure they could see my thumb was sticking up. That car nearly runned me down.

We was both shivering and our hands was getting froze 'cause we didn't have no gloves. Ruby Rose kept saying, "I'm cold, I wanna go back. This isn't fun."

I told her, "Shut up, Ruby Rose, we can't go back. We'll get in big troubles if we go back. We gotta go to Philadelphia."

Another car come. I sticked up my thumb, but I didn't go out in the road. This time the car stopped. It was full of men, four men, they put down the window and ask us where was we going.

I told them, "Philadelphia. Could you ride us there?"

"That's too far. We could take you part way, we could take you to Jefferson."

The man that was driving said one of us should get in the front seat and one of us should get in the back seat. I said no, me and Ruby Rose was gonna set together. And we did, we set together in the back, and one of the men in back had to go set in front.

It was a real old car, it was a clanky car, we go bumping up the road. Radio on real loud, and the men was talking another language, a different language from English language. They had beer, too, they was drinking out of beer bottles. I didn't like them. I didn't like that I couldn't understand what they was saying to each other.

"Are you talking French?" I ask them.

"Spanish. Want some beer?"

"No." They asked Ruby Rose, she said no, too.

The man who was driving, he said, "Where you girls from?"

"Back there. The town," I told him.

"You got family in Philadelphia?"

"Yes."

"You married?" Too many questions.

"No. But I got a boyfriend."

They all laughed when I said that, thought it was funny. I was just wishing we'd get to the town soon, I was just wishing to get away from them. Then the car stopped. But I couldn't see no town. We was in the woods.

"We're in the woods," I said.

The man that was driving said, "Well, you got no hurry, let's take a little walk now we're here."

"I don't want to take no walk. I'm cold."

"I could keep you nice and warm. Let your girlfriend wait in the car, she won't be alone." The other men laughed some more. I was feeling real scared and Ruby Rose was setting there biting on her hand. The man got out of the car, he come around to the back door, said, "Take off your glasses, I bet you look pretty without them glasses."

"I'm not taking off nothing."

"I just want for you and me to take a little walk. I'm not gonna hurt you. Then I'll take you to Jefferson."

I had to think if I should go or if I shouldn't go. Could be he wouldn't drive us no more if I didn't go. Or could be he would drive us. Who knows? I told Ruby Rose to stay there, told Ruby Rose I was coming right back, and I went with the man. It was so dark I couldn't even see where we was going. I tripped over something and he grabbed hold of my hand.

"Don't grab hold of my hand."

"What's the matter, don't you like men?"

"I wanna go back. I'm going back to the car now."

"First you gotta give me a little kiss." And he pushed his

face right in my face. I pushed it right back away, told him, "Stop it!" Told him, "I had enough, now I'm going back to the car!"

"Oh no," he said, and he grabbed my coat.

Bam. I kicked him right in his privates. Then I start running back to the car fast as a little bunny rabbit.

He come running along behind me, he was cussing and swearing. I heard the radio, they was still playing it, and that's how I could find the car. When I opened the door, the light come on inside and I seen Ruby Rose. She was in there kissing with one of the other men.

"Cut that out, Ruby Rose!" I pulled her out of the car and she come bump on the ground. The man that was trying to kiss me, he jumped in the car, he was still cussing like anything, he started up the car and they go bumping and clanking away. The back door was still open, they didn't even close up the back door.

"Why did they do that?" Ruby Rose said. "Why did they leave us here?"

"Shut up," I told her.

"I'm scared." She was laying on the ground, she was crying. I set down next to her. I was scared, too. All I could see was only woods and black places.

"I hear noises," she said. "I hear animals coming."

"We gotta start walking."

"Are we lost?"

"What do you mean, lost?" We was lost, but I wasn't gonna tell her that.

We start walking, walking up the road the same way the car went. It was a little road. Sometimes it was hard to see in the dark, I bumped right into a tree, didn't see it standing there.

"Why was you kissing with that guy?" I ask Ruby Rose.

" 'Cause he told me to."

"What's the matter with your brains? Don't you know no better?"

"I thought he liked me. Why does boys kiss girls except if they like them?"

"They don't like you," I told her. "They only want you for one thing, just one thing, that's how boys is. Except Thomas. I don't think he wants one thing."

Oh, we was cold. Shivering and teeths chatting, got our coats buttoned up to the top, but it didn't help much. My hands was froze, my legs was froze, even my nose was froze. I had an earache. Ruby Rose wasn't crying no more, just walking along holding my hand.

The little road come to a big road and then we was out of the woods. I saved us. We was lost and I saved us.

Ruby Rose wanted to get a ride in another car, but I told her, "Oh no, we're gonna walk." Anyway, I could see lights up the road. Must be it was a town. We had to go real slow for Ruby Rose, had to stop so she could rest a couple times. When we got closer we could see it wasn't no town up there, just only two places. A gas station and a diner. I told Ruby Rose, "Well, at least we could go inside, get ourselfs warm."

There wasn't nobody in the restaurant but the lady behind the counter. We set at one of the tables and looked at the menu.

"I'm cold," I told the lady when she come to our table. "I want something warm."

"How about some soup?" she said.

"Okay, give me some soup, please. And some tea."

"Me, too," Ruby Rose said. "Soup and tea."

"What kind of soup?" the lady ask.

I never ordered by myself before. How are you supposed to know what kind of soup they got? On the menu all it said was a cup of soup and a bowl of soup. Do you ask the lady?

"Bowl," I said. "I want the bowl."

"Are you girls trying to be funny?"

"Chicken soup," I said real fast. "We both want chicken soup."

We set there rubbing our hands, our ears, trying to get warm. Our noses was running, too. The lady brung us our tea first and we start in sipping it even while it was too hot.

"I didn't see no car drive up," the lady said.

"We don't have no car," I told her. "We was just out walking."

The lady didn't talk to us much after that, could be she thought we was peculiar 'cause we didn't have no car. She set by the counter and looked at a magazine while we ate up our soup. Sometimes she looked at us. Soon as we was done she come over with the check.

"You gotta leave now," she said. "I'm closing."

The check was a dollar forty. I took two dollars from my coat pocket and give it to her and she give me some change from the cash register. I pretended to count it, look like I know how much we're suppose to get back, but really I need to figure out that kind of stuff on paper.

We got another ride, but this time it was with two ladies and a little boy in the back seat, sleeping. I wasn't getting in no more cars with men, I learned my lesson. The ladies let us off in town. I don't know if it was Jefferson, didn't ask them where we was. There was red and green lights across the street, shining for the holidays, but no lights in the stores. Everything looked to me to be all closed up. We was both real tired. Had to go to the bathroom, too. We went behind a bush, first Ruby Rose, then me. Wasn't no one on the streets to see us, anyway.

Then, a real big problem. Where was we gonna sleep? Too cold to stay out all night, we would freeze up and die.

"Let's sleep in one of them cars," Ruby Rose said. That was a good idea she had. I told her so, too.

The first car we tried didn't open up, but the second car we tried did open up. I got in front and Ruby Rose got in back. We took our coats off, more comfy for sleeping, put them on top of us to keep warm. But still I was freezing. If I pulled my coat up to keep my top warm, then my feets was cold; if I pulled my coat down to cover my feets, then my top was cold.

I tried hard to forget how cold I was, tried hard to go to sleep, but all I could think about was the institution. That I sure rather be there now, I sure rather be in the institution. At least it's warm and got blankets. I was thinking, well, maybe running away wasn't such a good idea of mine, or maybe we should of waited for summertime. I was thinking about Philadelphia, too, what was it like. I did know it was a big city. I bet they got a lot of crime in Philadelphia.

Ruby Rose was sound asleep. Nothing bothers that girl when she wants to sleep. I tried to fold myself up little, make myself real small, so the coat could cover all of me. I guess I fell to sleep then.

What woke me was someone yelling.

I couldn't even remember where the heck I was, thought I was back in my own bed. Then I open my eyes, seen I wasn't in my bed, I was in a car. It was morning time. A man was standing by the car yelling, "Come out of there, come out of there!"

"I don't have to! Go away!" I yell right back at him. Ruby Rose was awake, the man woke her up, too. I told her, "Don't worry, he can't get in, I locked the doors last night."

Then he give up yelling, he walked away.

"Let's get out of here," Ruby Rose said, " 'cause maybe he's gonna come back."

When he turned the corner we jump out of the car, get our coats on and go real fast away from there. Go fast as we can up the street till we was sure he wasn't behind us. Till we was safe.

"Now we gotta get us some breakfast," I told Ruby Rose. So we walked some more, looking for a restaurant, a place to eat and warm up and go to the bathroom. And we seen one of them White Tower restaurants across the street.

"Wait a minute," I said. "Uh-oh." I had my hands in my

pockets trying to get them warmed and all of the sudden I thought, where's the money? I wasn't feeling the money no more.

"Ruby Rose, where's the money?"

"In your pocket."

I wiggle my fingers around in my pocket, wiggle and wiggle some more, come up with a quarter.

"Where's the rest of it?" Ruby Rose asked.

"I don't know. It's all gone. My money and your money."

"Somebody must of robbed us."

"Nobody could rob you if you don't know it," I hollered.

"There's some policemen, maybe they could help us find our money."

She was right, two policemen was coming up the street. Coming right at us. I wanted to run, but it was too late. What the heck. So what if they catch us, send us back?

"Are you the girls that was sleeping in the car?" one of them asked us. I thought, oh no, that man went and ratted on us.

"Yes," I said.

"Well, you better come with us."

Up the street was their police car. They told us get in, they told us they was taking us to the police station. Ruby Rose started to cry 'cause she thought they was gonna put us in jail. I didn't know if they could do that, put us in jail. I wonder how that man knew it wasn't our car?

One of the policemen turned around, asked me, "What's your name?"

"Winifred."

"What's your friend's name?"

"Ruby Rose."

"You're from the institution at Corona, aren't you."

"Oh no, we're not."

"Yes, you are. We got a warning about you, give us your names and said one was tall and one was cripple."

That shut me up.

When we got to the police station, they took us into a room to talk to another policeman. This one was setting at a desk and he looked to me to be real important. He told us to set down in the chairs. I thought I better act real polite. I said, "How do you do?"

"What's your name?"

"Winifred."

"Winifred Sprockett?"

"Yes."

"Is that Ruby Rose Seigler?" Ruby Rose was still crying and chewing on her hands.

"Yes. She's my friend. I don't hit her and she knows it, too."

"You girls run away from Corona last night, didn't you."

"Yes."

"Why did you run away?"

"'Cause I was sick of the whole darn institution. I wasn't trying to do nothing bad, I just wanted my freedom."

"Okay, Winifred. Take your friend and go wait in the other room."

Another policeman took us to a big room. It had benches and a little Christmas tree and pictures and signs all over the walls. There was a long desk with more policemen behind it. They told us to set on a bench.

"They're gonna put us in jail!" Ruby Rose kept saying. I never seen her so scared before. I didn't know if they was gonna put us in jail or if they wasn't gonna put us in jail, only thing I knew was I had to go to the bathroom. Real, real bad. I ask one of the policemen if they had a bathroom, he told me wait a minute. Then in comes a policeman lady to take us to the bathroom. Didn't want to let us go by ourselfs, must be they thought we was gonna run away again. That shows how smart they are. I had enough of running away.

When we got back to the bench, Ruby Rose started crying again. I told her, "You're a big cry baby. I never should of took you."

One of the policemen, he had a real friendly face, he come over and told Ruby Rose, "If I get you some coffee, would you stop crying?"

"She don't drink coffee," I told him. "She drinks tea. With sugar. I drink tea with sugar, too."

"We only got coffee or soda, so take your pick."

We picked coffee. He brung it to us in paper cups and he set down with us. The coffee had lots of milk and sugar in it and I drunk mine right up. It made me feel a little warm inside, I was still all froze up. Ruby Rose stopped crying and drunk up her coffee, too.

"So what was you two hobos doing out all night?" the policeman asked me.

"Trying to get to Philadelphia."

"Don't they treat you good at Corona?"

"Sometimes. But sometimes they don't."

"How long you been there? A long time?"

"Since 1938. July."

"That's a long time," he said. "That's a real long time."

I ask him, "Are you gonna put us in jail or are you gonna send us back to the institution?"

"Do you wanna go to jail?"

"No!"

"Okay. Then we'll send you back to the institution."

Ruby Rose said, "Thank you."

In a little while two more policemen come in the door. The nice one, the one that was talking to us, he said, "Your car's here, ladies," and he told the other two policemen, "These is the ladies that's waiting to go to Corona." He called us "ladies."

The policemen told us to come with them, and we was just out the door when the nice policeman come running after us. He got a whole bunch of candy canes in his hands, red and white stripey candy canes. "Wait a minute," he told us, "I got a present for you." He give us each a bunch of candy canes.

I said, "Oh, that's real nice of you, oh, what a lot of

candy canes!" Ruby Rose just took her candy canes and got in that police car real fast. You could tell she was in a big hurry to get away from there.

The nice policeman waved bye-bye to us. He called out, "You take care of yourselfs, okay?"

"We will!" I called back. I felt like I almost didn't want to leave him. I felt like he was a friend to me.

The policemen drove us all the way back to the institution, turned the heat way up so it was real warm in the car. I was still feeling cold way down in my bones. Coughing, too. I catched a cold from sleeping in a car.

I knew we was gonna be in real bad troubles when we got back to the institution, but I was glad we didn't get to Philadelphia. Too much crime there. Somebody could of killed us.

32

Our punishment was getting sent to the Behavior Center, the jail. For a month.

I done bad things before, but never so bad to get sent there. That's where they put you if you beat up an attendant, something terrible like that. Or run away. Most of the girls that gets put there is the real mean ones or the real disturbed ones.

The little room had a cot for sleeping and nothing else. There was a window with bars in it.

"Wait there," the attendant said when she put me in the room. "I'm coming right back." Wait there, where the heck did she think I was going?

She come back with scissors.

"You know what happens to girls who run away, don't

you?" She was smiling, but she had a nasty look in the eyes. I give her that nasty look right back. "Girls who run away get all their hair cut off."

"So what," I said.

"Stand up," she told me, and she cut the band out of my hair and snip, snip, snip, she goes with the scissors. Like when I was six years old, first come to the institution. I cried then, but I wasn't gonna cry for her. Just stood there, didn't say a peep, all the while she was cutting off my hair.

"How do you like that hair style?" she ask me. I wanted to tell her, "None of your beeswax," but I didn't. "I bet you'll never run away again," she said and she went out, locked the door behind her.

I felt my head. Wasn't hardly nothing up there. Not even as much hair as a boy has. I set back down on the cot. My hair was all over the floor, she didn't bother to clean it up. It looked pretty, and some of it got a cute little curl to it. I wished I could pick up all them pieces and tatch it back onto my head.

When supper time come, another attendant brung me a tray. All that was on that tray was a bowl of soup, a piece of bread and got butter on it, a glass of milk. I told her, "That's not a supper, that's a lunch."

She said, "Quit complaining and eat it 'cause that's all you get until breakfast."

"But that's not fair, I'm hungry!" Boy, was I hungry. Didn't have nothing to eat that day but candy canes.

I set on my cot and ate, ate every bit of food and nearly ate the tray, too. When I was done, my stomach was still making hungry noises.

When the attendant come back to get the tray, she asked did I want to go to the bathroom. I said yes. She took me out, down the hall. We passed lots of other locked-up rooms, but I couldn't tell which one Ruby Rose was in. The attendant come in the bathroom with me just like the policeman lady done. She ask me, "So what are you doing in here?"

"Making wee-wee."

She bust out laughing. I said, "What's so funny?"

"I was asking why you was in jail," she told me. And kept on laughing. But I got even. I didn't tell her.

The girl in the room next to me was a screamer. Started up after supper and kept going almost all the night. I could hear her scream and curse, sometimes she was calling for her mommy, sometimes she was calling for other people, and saying awful words. Banging at the walls, too. I laid on my cot and tried to sleep, but I couldn't. The noise was most terrible.

Next morning I hear someone unlocking my door and it was the first attendant, the one who cut my hair.

I told her, "I can't sleep. Make that girl be quiet, she screams all night."

She said, "This isn't no hotel, honey," and she took me down to the bathroom, told me I could get a shower. She took away my skirt and blouse, said, "You'll get your stuff back when you get out of jail." She give me something else to wear, a big gray dress. When I come back to the room my hair was gone from the floor. Must be someone come in and sweeped it up.

All day I set on the cot. I asked the attendant, "Can't I even have a book to read?"

"Honey, you can't have nothing."

So what else was there to do but set? Look around the room. The floor was gray, the walls was gray, the cot was gray and got white sheets and a dark-colored blanket. I counted the bars on the window, there was four. I counted the cracks on the walls, there was eleven. I bit my nails.

Sometimes I looked out the window. From my window I could only see a teeny bit of the driveway and the back of Lake Building. I stood at the window watching the snow coming down till my legs was tired. I could see a few girls going here, going there. I think I seen Mrs. Knopf, too.

The girl in the next room screamed half the day, half the night. Screaming for someone to let her out of the room, screaming for her mommy to come, screaming dirty words. My nerves was getting real bad and it was giving me a headache, all that racket. My cough was getting bad, too. Sometimes I cough so much it felt like my head was going bang, bang, bang, then I gotta go lay down on my cot.

The only people I could see or talk to was the attendants. Most was nasty, but this one attendant, she was nice. Whenever I yelled to go to the bathroom, she would come and let me out. The others, they didn't care if you go on the floor, they only take you when they're good and ready. But after a few days I was so sick of being alone I was even glad to see the nasty ones.

"My cough is getting worse," I told the attendant who cut off my hair. "I need some cough medicine." She just put my supper tray down on the cot and went back out, locked the door. A sandwich. Soup or sandwich, that's all they ever give you for supper.

When she come back to get the tray, I ask her, "Did you bring cough medicine?"

She said, "You don't need no cough medicine."

I laid there all that night. Even when the girl in the next room wasn't screaming or banging, I still couldn't sleep. I was coughing too hard. My throat hurt, too.

"Merry Christmas," one of the attendants told me when she brung me my breakfast.

"Merry Christmas?"

"Today's Christmas."

"Today?" I thought, how could it be Christmas when I didn't even know it? It seemed to me just like all the other days.

I started to sleep a lot, even with all that racket. Slept in the daytime, slept in the nighttime—who could tell the difference, anyway? They keep the lights on all the time, it's always bright in there. Sometimes I wake up, don't even know if it's day or night, have to turn around and look out the window to tell. And when they bring me my tray I wasn't always sure what I was getting, lunch or supper, 'cause I didn't know the time of day. Breakfast I could tell 'cause I always got some kind of cereal.

"I'm sick," I told the attendant who cut off my hair.
"What's wrong?"
"My cough, my throat, my chest. Can't even eat, my throat hurts so bad."
"You look okay to me, honey."

Sometimes I wake up and look at the bars. Looks like they're moving, going back and forth, going up and down. The cracks in the wall look like a scary monster. I try not to look at the cracks.
Sometimes I wake up and think I'm still in the car, shivering, can't get warm. My teeths is chatting.
The attendant said, "Why didn't you eat your supper?"
I said, "I'm sick. Get me help, please get me help!"
She took the tray away.

I opened my eyes, I felt something on my chest. A doctor was there, he was listening to my heart with one of them things that hangs from doctors' necks. I told him, "I'm so thirsty. Please could I have a drink?"
He said, "Wait a minute, you could have a drink in a minute." He ask me to open my mouth all the way up, looked in there with a little light, looked in my eyes and ears, took my temperature. He told the attendant, "She has to go to the hospital."

First I'd be cold all over, pull up all the blankets. Then I'd be hot all over, didn't even want the sheets. They give me shots, they give me medicine, they give me things to drink. They said I had pneumonia.

Sometimes I had crazy dreams. Then I'd wake up and think I'm still in that car, or in the Behavior Center, have to look around to see where I am. I woke up one time 'cause I thought the girl in the next room was screaming again, but the screaming was coming out of me. The nurse held my hand.

I wondered, did Gladys know I'm sick? Or maybe she was still in Baltimore.

Once I open up my eyes and seen Mrs. Knopf standing there in her coat and hat, she was just looking down at me. I wanted to tell her hello, but I was feeling too tired to talk.

My chest hurt, and when I breathed there come a funny noise, and that's what scared me the most. I know Jeannie got pneumonia, then she got all better, but my father got pneumonia and he died with it.

I ask the nurse, "Am I gonna die?"

She said: "What are you talking about? You're not gonna die."

I laid there and thought about what it would be like, what dying would be like. I do know you go up to heaven. No more tears, you be with the angels and the Virgin Mother, you do God's work for Him. But does it hurt? Did it hurt my father and mother when they died? All these things I wondered about while I was laying there. And I try very hard not to be so scared.

I open up my eyes again. The sun was shining in and standing by my bed was the Virgin Mother. It wasn't in a dream. It was in real. I seen her. She was wearing a white veil, got a blue and white cape around her, brown hair, just like in the pictures. I looked at her and she looked at me. Her face was sweet.

She said, "You're gonna be well and strong again."

I crossed myself, I said, "Thank you."

Then I fell to sleep and when I woke up she was gone.

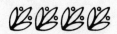

SUMMER
1959

33

Gladys sent me a big box of cookies in the mail, cookies she baked. Three different kinds. I took my cookies, took my book, went out to the front lawn. Had to pass Forest Building to get there and I seen Jeannie out in the yard. She was setting there in her wheeling chair fussing about something. You could tell she was feeling grumpy, so I didn't want to say hello to her. Sometimes I did go to see her when I got the time, when I wasn't working in the hospital, when I wasn't working for Mrs. Knopf. But she don't know what you're saying when you talk to her, so what's the use?

The summer was just starting, it was a beautiful day, green and sunny. Lots of the girls was out on the lawn. Girls setting on the grass together, girls walking around, girls waving to the cars. Everyone looked happy.

I set down under one of the trees where it was cool to eat my goodies and read my book. I had this book I got from Mrs. Knopf. It wasn't a library book, it was her book, I seen it on her desk while I was setting there answering the phone. It was wrote by a lady, a lady named Pearl Buck. Pearl Buck wrote lots of stories and this story was about she had a little mentally retarded child. Boy, was I ever surprised when I looked through that book and seen what it was about. I told Mrs. Knopf, "I didn't know a mentally retarded child could be in a book!"

"Anybody could be in a book, Winifred."

"Oh, could I borrow this book? Please?"

"That's real hard reading," she said. "I don't think you could read most of it." But she did let me borrow it.

It was a hard book. Lots of it I couldn't understand, too many big words, and no pictures. But I tried and tried and some parts I could read. The book told that the little child couldn't do the things the other kids was doing and that's how they could tell the little child was retarded. And told how much Pearl Buck loved the little child, even though she was retarded, and when the little child had to get put in an institution, Pearl Buck always come down to see her. It was a true story, too. I think Pearl Buck was a wonderful mother.

Sometimes Dr. Kravitz wanted to talk to me about my little girl life, ask me things about how did I get along with my family, what was they like. I told him Wanda had a sneaky look and my mother smacked me all the time.

I told him I remember when I was real little, like four or five, my daddy went to cut off the chicken's head and he fell down with his hatchet. The hatchet got stuck in the dirt. I was scared, I called, "Mommy, mommy!" She was around the side of the house, I think she was hanging the wash or something. She yelled back, "I'm busy, Winnie, shut up!" I said, "No! Mommy, mommy, daddy's on the ground!" And Patches was barking. She come running around to the back, said, "What's going on?" and then she seen my daddy laying on the ground. She run right into the house and called the ambulance and they took my daddy to the hospital. He had to stay there a long time. He had a heart attack, that's why he fell down. My mother told me, "You done the right thing by calling me, Winnie." She didn't smack me then. She praised me.

Sometimes she was nice to me. When she baked a cake. Me and Patches be out in the woods—we play tag out there, even play hide and seek together—and she would call me out the kitchen window. Then we come running, and she give me the bowl to lick out. That's the only time I ever hung around with my mother, when she was baking stuff. 'Cause she never give me no loving, she never took me in her arms and loved me.

Dr. Kravitz ask me why did I think my mother didn't love me. I told him, how should I know? Go ask my mother. I said, could be 'cause I wasn't her real kid. Or could be 'cause I was always carrying on.

Dr. Kravitz ask me why was I always carrying on. I told him when you carry on, people know you're there, boy, I told him sometimes it pays to carry on 'cause you get lots of attention. When you're good they don't notice you, but when you're bad they sure notice you. Don't have no choice about it.

I told Dr. Kravitz lots of things. But he can't tell nobody about it. It's the rules.

34

Mrs. McKenna, when she come down to visit Jeannie, took me home to visit for the week. More than my family done for me.

She give me Prudence's room to live in 'cause Prudence wasn't there. She went to college, then she went to France with her cousin. That room was beautiful, everything blue and white, a big bed and even a little table with a mirror and a seat to set on when you wanna look at yourself. White rug on the floor, you don't even want to walk on it 'cause you're afraid you'll get it dirty. And everywhere pictures of horses. Horse pictures on the walls, horse pictures on the dresser, horse pictures by the mirror.

"You could tell Prudence really likes horses," I said.

"I made room for you in the closet, Winifred," Mrs. McKenna told me. "You could hang your stuff in there."

I put some of my stuff in the closet, some in one of the drawers. Prudence had a whole lot of clothes, dresses and skirts and blouses and shoes and coats. Her closet looked to me like a store.

I don't think the rest of the house changed much since I been there a long time ago, still got all them rugs and everything, but some of the furniture was different and there was a big shiny piano in the living room. Also lots of pictures of Prudence. Mrs. McKenna showed me the ones in the hall, three pictures of Prudence on the beach when she was a little girl, got a white dress on and long braids. And there was a big picture of Prudence on the piano, just the face. Yellow curls, pink lipstick, looked to me to be a real happy girl.

We had our supper on the patio, a porch outside with furniture. It was like a picnic to eat out there with the trees and flowers and birds. Mrs. McKenna told me she wished she could of brung Jeannie home, too, said she just can't carry her around no more, can't lift her. Jeannie's too big.

I said, "Well, I sure am glad you brung me."

After supper she helped me call up Gladys to tell her where I was 'cause Gladys don't live all that far from the McKennas'. Twenty or thirty miles, I think. Mrs. McKenna called information, asked for the number of Clayton Oster in Hollis Falls, please.

Gladys was surprised to hear me on the phone. I never called her before. She said, "Winnie, is that you?" then she said, "Winnie, is anything wrong?" I laughed, told her no, told her I was at the McKennas' and maybe she could come see me 'cause it wasn't such a long drive. She said sure she could. She ask me to give her the phone number so she could call me back tomorrow.

I went to bed early. Couldn't wait. I got my book from the bag and jumped into Prudence's bed, but I didn't even want to read. Just wanted to lay there and look at that beautiful room. I felt like a queen in there. I thought, if I was Prudence I wouldn't go to no college, wouldn't go to no France, I would just stay here with Mrs. McKenna and live in this room.

In the morning Mrs. McKenna took me to town to get a bathing suit, 'cause I didn't have no bathing suit. I got a pretty green one, with white flowers, and after lunch we went to the pool. The McKennas belong to the pool—it's like a club—and you can't swim if you don't belong to the pool. They wouldn't even let you in the gate.

Mrs. McKenna set down with some ladies, but not me, I go running right over to that pool. It was my first time in a pool. I promised Mrs. McKenna I would stay in the low part, the part that wasn't deep, 'cause I can't swim. I hop right in that water, made a big splash. Oh, it felt so cool and good to me. I set down on the bottom and still my head was sticked up out of the water, and that was so fun. I thought, boy, I could stay all day in this water! Winifred the fish.

There was some kids throwing a great big ball, having a game in the water with the ball, laughing and shouting. I wanted to play that game, too. I know how to catch balls good. So I set there real still, I was waiting, and soon as that ball fell down on the water near me, I grab it up. Told the kids, "I got the ball! Come and get it!"

They said, "Throw it here!"

"Nope, you gotta come get it!"

"You better give that ball back to us!" they yelled. They was getting mad. I don't know why they was getting mad, I wasn't being mean.

"Okay, here's your darn ball," I said, and I threw it. Right into the deep part.

One of the little girls started crying and a lady come running to the side of the pool, ask the little girl, "What happened?"

"She took our ball," the little girl said, "and she wouldn't give it back. She threw it in the deep part."

"Don't blame me, it's not my fault," I told the lady. "I was just trying to play with them!"

Mrs. McKenna come running over to the side of the pool, too, talked to the lady a minute, then she said, "Winifred, come on out of the pool now and set with us."

"That's okay by me," I told her. "I don't even want to stay in this rotten pool no more."

The lady swimmed into the deep part to get the kids' ball for them, and I set at the table with Mrs. McKenna and her friends. They was playing cards. I read my book and drank sodas. When it come time to go home I told Mrs. McKenna, "I don't like this place, I don't want to come back here. And anyway, I think I'm getting a sunburn."

After we got back to the house—we was out on the patio—Gladys called. Mrs. McKenna went in to answer the phone, talked a little bit, then she called me in. Gladys told me she was coming Friday and Miriam was coming with her. Friday at two o'clock. I said, "Goody, goody!"

Mrs. McKenna took me on a picnic. We made ham sandwiches, put fruit punch in the thermos bottle, and go to have our lunch in the park. There was tables by the lake, that's where we set, and I did enjoy that so much. When I was done eating I said to Mrs. McKenna, "I'm gonna take my shoes off!"

I pull off my shoes and socks and go running on the grass in just my barefeets. Mrs. McKenna set at the table and laughed to see me having so much fun, said, "Be careful what you step on!" I just kept running back and forth. It tickled on the grass, and when the air hit my feets it give me a good feeling. I love to go barefooted. The heck with shoes.

Then we went for a walk around the lake to look for ducks 'cause we packed some extra bread for them. Everything was so pretty, little children playing with each other and people looking all happy to be out in the fresh air and sunshine. We walked and walked but didn't find no ducks. Then Mrs. McKenna said, "Winifred, look!"

A swan, a big white swan, was floating in the lake. I tried to throw it bread, but it was too far away.

I read in a fairy tale once about an ugly ducky that grew up to be a beautiful swan. I wonder where do swans go in the winter?

On Friday we went to town to get refreshments. Such as cheese and crackers, fruit and soda. After lunch I go upstairs, washed my face and hands, put on the nicest dress I got with me, set down by Prudence's mirror and comb my hair real neat. Then I went downstairs and set in the hammock on the patio to wait for my sisters to come.

They had Hannah and Marina with them. Only first I didn't know who them kids was, they got so big. I hug and kiss Gladys, hug Miriam and the kids, but the kids was shy, didn't hug me back. I made introductions, told Mrs. McKenna who was who, but I made a mistake. Said Hannah was Marina and Marina was Hannah.

"No, Winnie," Gladys said, "the one with the red hair is Marina." But it wasn't my fault, I got them mixed up 'cause Marina was bigger than Hannah even though she was the youngest.

Mrs. McKenna showed them the house, took them to see all the rooms and the pictures of Prudence, then she took them out to the patio to set. The kids got the hammock. When Mrs. McKenna went back inside to get the refreshments I went to help her, and Miriam come, too. She told me, "Winnie, I want to talk to you. Could we go in the living room?" I said sure.

"Winnie, I got something to tell you that's gonna make you very sad. Gladys is sick with cancer."

I said, "What?" I said, "Say that again."

So she said it again. And then she said, "Gladys don't know about it, she just thinks she has stomach problems."

"Miriam, is she gonna die?"

"I think so."

"But when?"

"I don't know, Winnie."

I felt so terrible I didn't know what to say after that, and you could tell Miriam felt real terrible, too.

"Winnie, are you okay?"

"I'm okay. I'm not gonna cry, don't worry."

"Well," Miriam said. "This sure is a nice house."

I said, "Yes, it sure is."

"Let's go back out now. Tell Gladys she looks good, 'cause she's failing."

Miriam went outside, but I went into the kitchen. Mrs. McKenna was in there cutting up some cheese. I whisper to her—I was scared Gladys or the kids might come in—I whisper, "Mrs. McKenna, Miriam says Gladys has cancer."

She put down her knife, she look at me, she said, "Oh no! Oh, dear!"

"I'm afraid I'm gonna lose her, Mrs. McKenna," I said, and the tears start to come. Mrs. McKenna set down at the table.

"Does Gladys know?"

"No."

"Oh dear," she said again. Then she told me, "Winifred, go in the bathroom and wash your face 'cause you can't let her see you upset. You gotta do your best to hide your feelings for a little while."

So I did, I did wash my face, then I went back outside. Mrs. McKenna come out with the refreshments and we all ate cheese on little crackers and the kids had watermelon. Then Mrs. McKenna told the kids where the strawberries was growing in back, 'cause they looked real bored, and they went to pick some.

I said to Gladys, "Oh, Gladys, you're looking pretty."

"I am?"

"Yes, you look so good." But she didn't. I could see she was getting thin in the face.

After awhile the kids come back with their hands full of strawberries, pop some in their mother's mouth, pop some in Miriam's mouth.

"They sure do taste good," Gladys said. "I'd like to get me some more. Could you show me where they're growing, Winnie?"

So Gladys and me walk down the little path behind the house, and when we get to the strawberries she said, "Winnie, I wanna come see you again before something's gonna happen to me."

"What do you mean? Nothing's gonna happen to you."

"Oh yes," she said. "I got something wrong with me and they won't tell me."

She did know. But I didn't tell her.

We picked some strawberries. I couldn't talk, I was trying too hard not to cry. When we get our hands full of strawberries, we start back up the path.

"Miriam will look after you," Gladys said. "I'm gonna make her promise."

"Okay," I said.

When we got back, Mrs. McKenna got paper cups to put all the strawberries in so the kids could take them home. Gladys didn't even eat any. The kids was talking about how they was ready to go home and Gladys told Miriam she was feeling real tired now.

"I think we better go now, Winnie," Gladys said.

I walked them to the car, I kissed them good-bye, and they left. Miriam was driving.

And that's the last time I ever seen Gladys.

Then I really did cry, broke down and cried. Mrs. McKenna told me I should try not to be so upset. Mrs. McKenna said maybe Gladys wouldn't die, said you never could tell with cancer.

"You gotta pray, Winifred," she said. "Maybe your prayers will be answered."

"They never was before!"

"Maybe you never prayed hard enough. Pray for Gladys every day. Who knows what's gonna happen?"

Mr. McKenna come home that night. He was in Chicago doing his business, then he took an airplane and a taxi cab to get back. We was all supposed to go to a restaurant for supper, but I heard Mrs. McKenna say, "Well, maybe we shouldn't go now, maybe Winifred's too upset."

"Go up and see how she's feeling," Mr. McKenna said, and Mrs. McKenna come up. I was laying on Prudence's bed.

"Are you okay enough to go out for supper?" she ask me.

"Yes," I told her, "I feel better. I been doing a lot of praying."

When we come home from the restaurant, I had to pack my stuff. I was going back to the institution on Saturday. Mrs. McKenna helped me pack, then she had to pack, too, and so did Mr. McKenna, 'cause after they drove me to the institution they was going on a vacation together.

Before I went to bed Mrs. McKenna come in to set with me a little. "Think good thoughts," she told me. "Sometimes that makes good things happen."

"Thanks, Mrs. McKenna. I'm gonna try."

I could hear them talking real quiet in their room and soon I fell to sleep.

35

Every Sunday I go to church in the Assembly Hall, don't skip it like I sometimes use to. And I pray, 'cause I know if you pray with the rosary and say your Hail Marys, you're talking to the Virgin Mother.

I told her, "Please don't take Gladys away from me, please make Gladys all better like you made me all better." I told her, "I know you got lots of things to do, you can't answer all the prayers, but please answer this prayer."

Mrs. McKenna sent me some postcards from their vacation, then a couple weeks later she sent me a package. I open it and inside was a Bible, white with gold on the sides. It was the most beautiful book I ever seen in my life.

I could have. Boris, don't be silly." Avery opened the
glove compartment. "I hope." He gave a little laugh. "Any
roll film.... You won't tote of under to the very least,
answer all the crying telephones, you to this busy
time... Sylvania sent me some powerful Republican
over their computers. On the nathan's in the large
corporate and make any sophisticated. When we're coming? The
is that the most hardball your power spoken any last

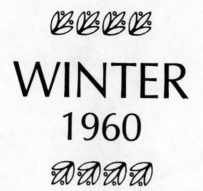

WINTER
1960

36

When Miriam come to tell me Gladys died I was real surprised to see her, couldn't hardly believe my eyes when I walked into Mrs. Demerest's office and there she was. I thought, what the heck is she doing at the institution? I didn't think maybe Gladys died. I just got a letter from Gladys before Christmas and she told me she was feeling a little better, starting to put some meat on her bones. Also sent me a pretty sweater for my Christmas present. And a Merry Christmas card from the kids.

Mrs. Demerest went out of the office when I come in so me and Miriam could be alone. I thought, "Uh-oh, must be something's wrong."

"Gladys died, Winnie."

"What?" That's all I could say.

"She died two weeks ago."

The phone started ringing on Mrs. Demerest's desk. Miriam went to the door to look for her, then the phone stopped ringing so she come back.

"But she sent me a Christmas present!"

Miriam didn't say nothing, and then I bust out in tears.

"It's better for her this way," she said. "She had a lot of pain."

In a little while Mrs. Demerest come in with a box of tissues. I blowed my nose, wiped my eyes.

"Did you have the funeral already?"

"Yes."

"But why didn't you tell me? Why couldn't I go to her funeral?"

"We was scared to take you, Winnie, we knew how upset you was gonna be. We was scared you might do something crazy."

"You should of took me! You should of took me, you should of took me, you should of took me!"

"Stop it, Winnie!"

"Come on, Winifred," Mrs. Demerest said, "we're gonna put you to bed now." She and Miriam got my arms and made me come upstairs with them, all the while I was yelling. And then Miriam was gone and Mrs. Demerest and Mrs. Potts made me get in my bed, didn't even take off my dress, and Mrs. Demerest said, "We're gonna get you a shot, help you calm down a little."

"They should of took me! They should of took me!" I kept screaming. "I wasn't gonna jump in the grave!"

I wouldn't stay in bed. I stood up all night and I cried softly. The night attendant told me, "Go back to bed. I got orders to keep you in bed."

"Gladys died," I told her. "My sister Gladys died."

"So what do you expect me to do about it? Get back in your bed."

For days they kept me in bed. I cried, wouldn't talk to nobody, wouldn't eat, wouldn't take my medicine. They sent Dr. Kravitz to me. He said, "I'm sorry to hear what happened to you about your sister."

"Nobody else could ever be like Gladys to me, nobody!"

"I know, Winifred, I know. But you better start taking your medicine, else you're gonna have a breakdown."

I did have a breakdown, I think. A breakdown is when you cry, do crazy things, say crazy things. I was laying in bed crying and talking to myself all the time. I say, "Am I gonna be all right?" then I tell myself, "No, I'm not gonna be all right!" Sometimes I jump out of bed, then they have to catch me, put me back in bed and give me a needle to make me sleep. I almost went crazy.

They put me in the hospital for a couple days where it was quiet, where they had more kinds of medicines to give me. I think Dr. Kravitz told them to do that. He come to see me in the hospital, he set and talked to me. He was trying to make me feel better, trying to make me come back to myself.

Mrs. Knopf come to see me while I was in the hospital, too. She brung me candy. A box of buttercreams. She said, "What a sad thing, Winifred. I'm so sorry for you."

"I was special to Gladys," I told Mrs. Knopf. "Now I can't be special no more."

37

I read my Bible a lot. My favorite thing is the Twenty-third Psalm which I read so much I could almost remember it.

Sometimes I think to myself, is there really a Virgin Mother? It comes back yes, always the answer comes back, "Yes, there is." There has to be a Virgin Mother, she's God's mother. So if she's God's mother, she's our mother, too. She's the one takes care of us.

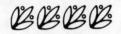

WINTER
1962–63

38

It was a happy day for Lucy, leaving the institution. We set around on our beds watching her pack. The institution even give her a real suitcase to put her stuff in.

Lucy said, "Boy, am I gonna have a ball!" She knew we was all feeling jealous, she liked that. "I'll go in town every day and go to the stores."

Her social worker come to get her before lunch, take her to the nursing home. We stood on the steps to wave bye-bye to her, called out, "Good luck!" "Have fun!" "Stay away from the men!"

I guess the institution puts the girls in nursing homes 'cause they want them to live in the community, but they don't have no private homes to send them to. Also, they want to get them out of the institution to make room for the girls that's waiting to come in. So they pick out which girls. It's according to reports about their behavior and their work and what their social worker says. Some of the girls come back to the institution, can't make it. But some of them never come back. They do okay in the outside world.

A social worker is someone who takes care of your case. She's your friend. The name of my social worker is Mrs. Handelman. She's not just my social worker, she belongs to some of the other girls, too. Mrs. Handelman has three grandchildren and she likes to show us their pictures. She comes to see us, talks, reads the reports about what good things we done, what bad things we done. Sometimes she takes us into town when we save up our money and we buy things such as deodorant, hair curlers, cigarettes, and magazines.

Always I ask Mrs. Handelman, "When will it come my turn to get out of the institution?"

She tells me, "Just keep trying to do good, Winifred, then we'll see." I was still getting into devilments sometimes, hit and holler, I get nervous and cry. But I can't help it, it's my nerves. My nerves tighten up, then I have to pull back away from them. I take pills twice a day, Dr. Kravitz give them to me. I was getting tired of taking pills twice a day, but if I don't take my medicine I get even more nervous. I'd give a million dollars if Miriam could find a doctor, a special doctor, to take my nerves away from me.

39

I only see Thomas every couple months when we're both on the list for the dance. He give me another picture of him, I asked him to, 'cause somebody stole the old one. It was getting all tore up from hanging on the wall so long, anyway. I give him a picture of me, too. One time when Gladys come to see me she brung her camera and took some pictures of me by my building. Then she got one of the attendants to take a picture of both of us together. She sent a couple of them to me. After Gladys died, I slept with the one of me and her under my pillow for a long, long time.

I like to tease Thomas, I do. I tell him I got another boyfriend and I make him mad.

He says, "No, you got no other boyfriend."

I say, "Oh yes, I do!"

He says, "I'll kill the man whoever takes you away from me."

He know I'm teasing, though, he teases me, too. Says he's got another girlfriend. I just tell him, "Oh, that's good. Is she nice like me?" He laughs, he says no.

Thomas run away from his aunt's house when he was a kid. When they catched him, they put him in Kortland.

We like to set together and talk. We don't dance too much, we like to watch the other people. Sometimes we don't even talk, just look at each other. Thomas has nice kind eyes, blue with glasses. I feel like he's talking to me with his eyes.

"You're looking sad," I tell him.

He tells me, "That's 'cause I'm always lonely for you, sweetheart."

"Well, we're inside the same boat. I miss you, too."

Only thing, Thomas isn't good-looking. He's tall like I am, real skinny, has gray hair with some white in it and a little black. His face is old. But looks don't count, he has personality. Besides, I don't class myself good-looking, neither.

When I'm at a dance and girls try to talk to me, I don't listen to them. I'm all wrapped up in Thomas. The girls call me man-crazy. But that's not true, I'm not man-crazy, I just like Thomas. He's different, you could practically say I know him. I feel sorry for him. When I'm with Thomas, anybody calls me I won't answer them. 'Cause I'm with Thomas. I want to spend time with Thomas.

I wonder if that's how love starts.

Dr. Kravitz's wife had a baby, a baby girl. Dr. Kravitz was real happy about it 'cause they only had boy kids, lots of boy kids. I told Dr. Kravitz if I ever get out of this darn place, maybe someday I might get married with someone. Don't even have to be Thomas, just a nice man with a nice personality, works hard, treats his parents good and don't bum around. It sure would feel different to be married, I would have my own home. I told Dr. Kravitz if I learn to cook, I think I could do it.

But then I'd have to do housework all the time. Sweeping up, dusting, mopping floors, making beds, wash the dirty clothes. And I hate housework. So maybe I wouldn't get married. 'Cause if I get married I couldn't travel and I want to travel, I want to travel to everywhere. Like Paris.

Whenever I talk about the future, Dr. Kravitz smiled. He liked it. I wasn't seeing him regular no more, only I go to him sometimes if I had a bad problem I couldn't work out for myself. He told me he'd always be there for me if I needed him. He told me a lot of my problems come from I was unwanted when I was a little child, kept telling me, Winifred, it's time to forget about the past, you gotta go into the future. I think that means you live, each day you live, and forget about what happened yesterday. Just worry about each day you're living and wait and see how things work out.

40

Mrs. McKenna come down to visit Jeannie a couple weeks after Thanksgiving and she stopped by my building, see if I wanted to come with her. I didn't want to go to Forest Building, but I didn't tell her that.

We visited Jeannie in the Day Room, an attendant brung her in. Couldn't go nowhere, it was cold and starting to rain. Jeannie just laid back in her wheeling chair playing with something she got in her hands, a toy or something. She didn't even seem to know her mother. Maybe that's 'cause Mrs. McKenna don't come as much as she use to come.

Mrs. McKenna talked to her a little, talked to her like you talk to a baby, and sometimes Jeannie smiled, sometimes she fretted. She wasn't nothing like pretty, she looked old with no teeths and even got some hair that was gray. Then Mrs. McKenna talked to a couple attendants, ask how was Jeannie getting along. I just set with Jeannie, didn't know what to say. In the corner one of the low-grades was setting on the floor taking all her clothes off.

"Do you wanna go have some coffee with me before I leave?" Mrs. McKenna ask me.

"Oh, I sure do!"

So we asked at Meadow and they said yes, Winifred could go, just have her back for supper. We went to the diner in town, the one Gladys use to take me to. I had tea and cake and Mrs. McKenna had coffee. She was in a diet.

She told me, "You're looking so grown up. I like your hair curled." I said thank you, gobbled down my cake.

"I should try to get down here more," she said.

"I don't think Jeannie minds," I told her. "She don't know the difference."

"No. She don't."

"At least you still come see her when you got time. A lot of families are ashamed when they got a little retarded child. A lot of families like to forget about the little child."

"Do you hear from Miriam?" Mrs. McKenna ask me.

"I'm going to her for Christmas. She invited me."

"Oh, isn't that real nice."

"She writes to me sometimes, too. I think Gladys made her promise."

Mrs. McKenna paid our check, then we had to go to the drugstore so she could get more cigarettes.

I was standing there looking at all the pretty stuff, the bubble baths and powders, when I seen Mrs. DePalma come in. She's an attendant from Grove Building, only she wasn't wearing her uniform, just got on slacks and regular shoes with her raincoat, and first I didn't recognize it was her. But she seen me.

"What are you doing here?" she said. Said it real loud, too. There was some other people in the drugstore, and a pretty lady with a dog. They all looked at me.

I said, "I didn't run away. I'm with my friend and she's getting cigarettes."

"Well, I'm gonna call the institution."

"So what, go ahead and call, they know I'm out. I'm with my friend."

"Oh, I bet you are!"

I march right over to Mrs. McKenna, said, "Mrs. McKenna, aren't you my friend?"

"What's the trouble here?" she said.

"Just checking up on Winifred. Sorry," Mrs. DePalma said. Said it real polite and friendly, not like she talked to me.

Mrs. McKenna told her, "Next time you do your checking up, do it a little nicer. Don't you know she got feelings same as everybody else got feelings?"

I was almost crying when we got in the car. "Why did she have to say it so loud, Mrs. McKenna?" 'Cause you're always afraid when you go into stores, afraid someone is gonna know where you come from.

Mrs. McKenna still looked mad. "I don't know, Winifred. She had no rights to do that."

I told her, "Well, if them people know where I come from, they can't do nothing about it, anyway. So let them talk. It don't bother me."

41

That's when Willy called me mentally retarded. When I went to Miriam and Willy's for Christmas.

They was fighting about me the first night. I guess they thought I was sleeping but I wasn't, and my bed was on the sofa in the living room, so I could hear every single darn thing they was saying. They was talking about Miriam wanted to invite some friends over on Christmas Eve, have drinks together with them. And Willy was saying no, wait until after Christmas and Miriam said, "I know why you don't want them to come. You don't want them to come 'cause Winnie's here." Willy said, "That's right, Miriam, I sure don't!"

And that's how I could tell Willy was ashamed of me.

In a little while he come downstairs. I told him, "If you don't want me here I'll be real happy to go back tomorrow, then you could have all your friends come over."

"What was you doing? Laying there listening?"

I said, "I got good ears." He went into the kitchen. When he come back through the living room, I told him, "I don't even like your house, I liked Gladys's house better. I wouldn't even come here if Gladys was still alive."

Next day, it was the day of Christmas Eve, Wanda and Kenneth and their boys come over. They use to live far away but they got jobs here so they could move back to where they was coming from. They are school teachers.

I didn't want to see Wanda again, she use to be so mean to me, always picking. I thought she was still gonna be picking. But she was nice, she was real friendly. Talk to me a lot, ask me about what I was doing at the institution, listened to me when I told her. Isn't that something how people could change like that? Still got that pretty face, but plump, she was near to the plump side. Kenneth was nice, too. Only I didn't like the bigger kid, his name was Kenny. He kept following me around, kept watching me. Then I heard him ask Wanda, "Why does Aunt Winnie talk funny?" Wanda said, "That's just how she is."

Miriam and Willy and Kenneth was in the living room. I

went in there, set down next to Miriam, ask her, "Miriam, do I talk funny? Kenny says I talk funny."

Kenneth heard me I guess, said, "Kenny shouldn't be saying things like that, it isn't right."

"It sure isn't. I know how to talk clear now. I had help, that's why I went to the institution, to get special help. And my nerves was bad."

"That's right, Winnie," Miriam said, "you was a real nervous kid. You sure needed lots of special help."

"Don't give her them lies about special help, Miriam," Willy told her. And he told me, "You didn't need nothing special. You're mentally retarded, that's why you went to the institution."

Kenneth said, "Willy, be quiet."

Boy, I wanted to bust Willy's mouth in. I hollered at him, "Who the hell is mentally retarded?" I hollered at him, "Not me!"

Miriam yelled at him too. Willy just got up, said, "Well, I'm sorry that had to come out," and he went upstairs. I run into the bathroom, didn't want no one to see me crying. Wanda was standing by the living room door. I know she heard what Willy said, too.

Christmas morning Miriam called Hannah and Marina to tell them Merry Christmas. They live in Baltimore now and Miriam really does miss them. Then we open our presents. They give me a manicure set, I was trying to grow my nails again. Every time I get them to growing, something happens to make me bite them off again. I give them little things to put salt and pepper in. They was puppy dog shape.

But it wasn't no fun. I was just waiting to go back to the institution tomorrow. I had enough of Willy.

42

I kept saying to myself, who's telling the truth and who isn't? I kept asking myself, am I mentally retarded? The answer always come back no, no you're not.

I ask Mrs. Knopf, "Am I mentally retarded?"

She said, "What made you ask a question like that?"

"Miriam's husband said I was, Miriam's husband said that's why I'm in the institution."

Mrs. Knopf was checking some of the kids' workbooks. She told me, "That was a mean thing for somebody to say to you."

"It sure was."

"The reason you come here, Winifred, is you needed training. Special training."

"And my nerves," I said. "My nerves is bad."

I give Mrs. Knopf her phone messages from the morning. I finish dusting the books and shelfs, took out the wastepaper basket. Then it was time for me to go to the hospital.

"I don't really care what Willy said," I told her. "I'm not worried about being mentally retarded no more, I just set and laugh about it."

My job in the hospital was to sort out the dirty linen and get the clean linen from the laundry. I really learn a lot of different things while I was working at the hospital, such as watching nurses change bandages and give medicine and shots. I wish I could be a nurse. Hospital work is very interesting. That is, if you think so.

While I was sorting out the dirty stuff, I was thinking about that book Pearl Buck wrote, that book about the little mentally retarded child. And I thought, hmmmmm, if Pearl Buck could write a book about a little mentally retarded child that went to an institution, maybe I could write a book about me being in an institution. Show people I got something upstairs, instead of nothing. Brains.

I told Mrs. Knopf, "I think I'm gonna write me a book."
  "A what?"
  "A book. Pearl Buck wrote about a little mentally retarded child. So why couldn't I write about me? That would show people and Willy I'm not retarded!"
  "You couldn't do it," Mrs. Knopf said.
  "I bet I could," I said. "You dare me?"
  "I dare you."
  Mrs. Knopf give me a notebook from the supply closet, a brand new one, and a pencil. She told me I could take them back to the building with me. Told me if I needed help with my spelling to just come to her. I ask her, "What should I name my book?"
  She said, "Well, what's it gonna be about?"
  "About my life in the institution."
  "Then that's what you should name it."

I started my book in the hospital. When there wasn't no more dirty linen to take care of, I wash my hands and set down on a pile of sheets. I could tell it was gonna be harder than I thought it was gonna be. How do you start off? Should I say, once upon a time? How do you know what to write and what not to write? On the front of my notebook I put, "'My Life in the Institution' by Winifred Sprockett" in my best handwriting.
  Well, I thought. What comes next?

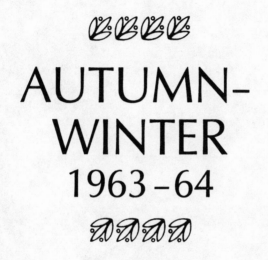

AUTUMN-
WINTER
1963 –64

43

In the summertime Mrs. Handelman told me I might get out of the institution, go to a nursing home.

I said, "When!"

She told me, "I'll see what I could do. I have to write letters. I'm trying to find you a place up near Miriam."

I thought I'd never get out, I had to wait and wait. But I didn't forget about it. Always I was thinking about it, that I might get out of the institution. That I really might get out.

I didn't even know I was going away until I started to get all my tests done. Me and Estelle Sampson and Dolly and some of the girls from Lake Building was on the front lawn waving to the cars. We wave and shout, "Hello!" and sometimes they will wave back at us. But when a man waves, the girls go all silly, start yelling stuff like, "Hi, loverboy!" calling for the men to come visit them. Then I just walk away, go find another thing to do.

Ruby Rose seen me on the front lawn and come after me, told me Mrs. Demerest was looking for me. I went back to Meadow and Mrs. Demerest told me to go right to the Psychology Department, they was waiting on me to get one of them I.Q. tests done. That's to see how much you know.

So I went and had my test and I didn't do too bad—tell about the pictures and do the blocks and answer the questions—but some of the stuff I didn't know. I know lots of things, but they didn't ask me those things so I didn't tell them.

Next day after breakfast they call me to come to the hospital to get a hearing test. I done pretty good on that one.

Still I didn't know something was going on until after a couple days Mrs. Demerest sent me back to the hospital to get a check-up, blood test, chest X-ray. And when they was done I had my teeths inspected. I ask the nurses, "Why am I getting all these tests?" They said, "We don't know."

When Mrs. Handleman told me she found a nursing home for me, when Mrs. Handelman told me I was leaving the institution, I didn't even believe it. If you're stuck in an institution so many years and someone tells you you're gonna get out of the institution, gonna be free, you don't know how to believe it. Your ears hear it, but I don't think your brain knows; it takes a few minutes for your brain to find out. Then, when your brain finds out, then you could start to believe a little bit.

"I'm leaving, Ruby Rose, I'm getting out of here!"

"How come?"

"'Cause Mrs. Handelman found me a nursing home, she found me a nursing home forty miles from Miriam's town."

"Are you going today?"

"No, Friday!"

"That's good," Kissy said. "Your mommy's coming for you."

Ruby Rose said, "I don't want you to go."

"Don't worry," Billie told her, "she'll be back."

"Oh no, I won't be back. I'm never coming back to this place!"

I had to go see Mrs. Knopf, tell her I was going away. That was the hard part, that was the part I didn't wanna do, tell

Mrs. Knopf good-bye. I think Mrs. Knopf understands just what kind of girl I am. We don't never fight, we get along just like mothers gets along with daughters.

She said, "I hope you're gonna be real happy, Winifred. And you send me lots of letters, let me know how you're making out."

"I will."

"What about the book, the book you're writing? Are you gonna take it with you?"

"No. I only done a few chapters anyway. I don't want to write about the institution no more, just only want to forget about it."

"Well, don't throw it out, give it to me. If you change up your mind, I could mail it to you."

"Okay, Mrs. Knopf. I gotta go back to my building now." I didn't have to go back to my building, I wanted to get away from Mrs. Knopf. I was feeling like maybe I was gonna cry.

I wish Mrs. Knopf was my real mom, I do.

I thought, hmmmm, should I say good-bye to Jeannie or shouldn't I?

Jeannie was out in the yard after supper, she was asleep in her wheeling chair. I tippytoed over and set down on the grass. She got on a long shirt and I could see her diapers peeping out. There was black and blues on her arms and legs. No shoes on the feets, they don't put shoes on the low-grades that can't walk. Only socks when it gets cold.

I set there watching Jeannie sleeping. I was thinking about how she looked when she first come to the institution. Blonde curls, such a pretty little face.

I whisper real quiet, "Bye, Jeannie."

Friday morning the attendants packed my things. The institution give me some clothes to take and stuff like a toothbrush and hairbrush and toothpaste. Give me a suitcase, too.

I took Thomas's picture down from the wall, put it in the suitcase. I had lots of stuff in my Belongings Box. Had to take everything out, put it all on my bed, figure out what I did want and what I didn't want. I packed my picture of Gladys and me. I packed my letters, I had some letters and birthday cards and Christmas cards I saved up for years and years, even a couple letters my daddy wrote me when I was a little girl. They was yellow and a little tore and you couldn't hardly read them no more, but still I wanted them. I packed my manicure set, my deodorant and the cold cream Thomas give me. Also my books, I had three books.

I give Ruby Rose the Archie comics and a hair ribbon and the comb I won when I was a bunny. I give Franny a pair of shoes Gladys buyed me a long time ago. They didn't fit no more, I wear a size 9½ now, but I didn't want to throw them out. They didn't fit Franny neither, too big, but she was glad to have them.

All the while I'm packing I'm thinking it's like a dream. My whole life I waited to get out of this place, now I'm getting out, but it don't seem real. Like it's in a dream. Or maybe April Fool.

"Don't forget about me," Ruby Rose said.

"I won't. I'm gonna write you."

"But I can't read good."

"I'll write with little words."

I got into the car and waved bye-bye to the girls. It was starting to feel real to me that I was going away, it was starting to feel real to me that I was gonna have a whole new life. It was starting to be such a big feeling of real that I was getting scared.

When we drove out the gates, Mrs. Handelman said, "Winifred, stop looking back. When you look back it means you're gonna come back." But I kept looking back.

44

Mrs. Handelman had coffee with Mrs. Tubber in the kitchen, then she said, "I gotta go now, Winifred."

"Couldn't you stay a little longer?"

Mrs. Tubber told her, "Winifred's feeling shy. I'm gonna take her around, introduce her to people, then she's gonna feel to home."

I ask Mrs. Handelman, "Will you come back to see me?"

"Sure I will. I'll be back next week, see how you're doing."

I didn't care to have Mrs. Tubber introduce me, just wanted to be alone so I could get use to the place without people looking. So Mrs. Tubber told a lady, a lady who was Caroline, to show me where was my room. Caroline was old with a cane and a big black sweater. It took a long time to get to the third floor 'cause she walked so slow, and my suitcase was heavy, too.

What a pretty room! Little purple flowers all over the walls, white curtains on the windows, and only four beds slept in there. There was four dressers, too.

Caroline said, "That's your bed and that's your dresser."

"My dresser? I got my own dresser?"

She said yes, she went back downstairs.

I laid on my bed. It had a cover on it, not just a blanket but a real cover. Bumpy, white, and pretty. I got up and looked out the windows. There was two windows and got them things like cranks, you turn the crank and the window opens up. Outside I could see apple trees. I love apple trees. They make me think of my home, my little girl home.

I went back to my bed, laid down again. I was tired.

After awhile I smelled food cooking, suppertime smells. Then I knew I was hungry. Still I stayed up there 'cause I didn't know what I was suppose to do, go downstairs all by myself or wait for someone to come get me. Then I thought, hmmmm, maybe I better go get my food, maybe if I wait there's gonna be nothing left for me.

While I was going down, I bump into a lady coming up. She said, "You're Winifred."

I told her, "I know."

"Well, I'm Bridey, I was just coming up to get you. It's suppertime."

So I went down with her. She was friendly, plump and old and sweet in the face. She showed me how to get my supper, you go to the kitchen, you get your plate from the lady. Then we went to the dining room and I set next to Bridey at one of the tables.

There was men there, too, not just ladies. And most of them old. Gray hair, wrinkled-up faces, that kind of old. Bridey told everyone at the table that this here's Winifred and she told me the people's names. But I couldn't remember them all, too many names.

I ate up all my food, took my plate back to the kitchen, wanted to ask the lady for seconds, but I thought maybe I better not. Mrs. Tubber was in there; she was eating her supper, too. She ask me, "Did you meet Maude yet?"

"Who's Maude?"

She took me to the dining room, took me over to one of the tables where a girl was eating. She was the only one who wasn't old, she looked to be about my age. Mrs. Tubber said, "Winifred, this here's Maude. Maude, this here's Winifred." Maude just kept eating, but she waved at me.

I watched a little television, then I went up and unpacked my stuff. Put my clothes in my dresser real neat, hung up my dresses in the big closet. I had three dresses. I put the other stuff, such as the books and manicure set and my hairbrush and cold cream, on top of the dresser. Then I laid down on my bed, read my Bible till the others come up. It was just like being a regular person.

Three ladies slept in my room with me, one of them was
Caroline. I ask somebody, "Do you do roll call here?"
"Roll call?"
"You know, to check if we're all in."
"No, we don't do no roll call."
I yelled, "Goody, goody, no roll call!"

My bed felt strange, different. I had troubles sleeping. And
all the night Caroline walked back and forth, back and forth
across the room, sometimes she stood and looked out the
window a long time. Every time I wake up I seen her going
here, going there, wearing her black sweater and bumping
things with her cane.
I ask her, "Don't you ever sleep?"
She said, "Sorry, honey, if I'm bothering you."
But it wasn't noisy. Nobody got the fits.

When I woke up in the morning time I thought I was in the
institution. But it was too quiet. Nobody yelling, no girls
fighting and teasing, no attendants talking loud. So then I
thought I wasn't in the institution. But I had to look around
a minute to remember what this place was. Then I seen the
windows, seen the cranks, remembered the apple trees outside, and I thought, oh boy, I'm out in freedom!
No one was in the beds, but a lady was standing by the
mirror, got real long gray hair, got hairpins in her mouth.
She was putting up her hair, she was sticking the hairpins in
her hair to hold it up. I laid there in bed a little while. It was
nice to watch her. I told her, "You got pretty hair."
She said, "That's 'cause I always took real good care of it.
You better get up, get dressed, you're gonna miss breakfast." She talked funny with hairpins in her mouth.
I hop out of bed, got my toothbrush, toothpaste, ask the
lady, "Do I take a shower now or bedtime?"
"It don't bother me none when you take a shower."

Some hairpins dropped out of her mouth when she said that. I didn't laugh.

After breakfast Mrs. Tubber said, "Why don't you take a walk with Maude? She could show you where the grocery store is." Well, that's something you sure can't do in the institution! But Mrs. Tubber had to ask Maude. I was shy of asking her.

Off we went, me and Maude, up the street past the pretty little houses. I run over to pet the big dog that was tied to one of the fences, a pretty dog, black and brown. It was a cool day, gray all over the sky, but it was a happy day. I was taking a walk, I was going to the grocery store.

I told Maude, "I think I'm gonna do this every day."

"Go to the grocery store?"

"Go everyplace. I wanna go everyplace. I might even travel someday."

"Can you drive a car?"

"No. But I could go on a plane. Or I could go on a train."

"I bet you don't have enough money for that. You need to buy tickets."

"So? I'm gonna get me a job soon."

In the grocery store they sold mostly stuff like bread and food, but they did have them big clips for the hair and I needed a clip to make a ponytail. I had some money, Mrs. Handelman said she was gonna make the State give me a little money every month, so I paid for my hair clip. But when it come time for Maude to pay, she couldn't find no money in her pockets. So I told her, "Don't worry, Maude, I'll buy you the bubble gum. I like to do good deeds."

It started raining on the way back. In the house it was cozy, the old people was setting around real quiet. They was watching television, playing cards, talking. Nobody hollering, nobody fighting, you could tell all of them people got along real well.

After lunch I went in the town with Mrs. Tubber. No-body else wanted to go 'cause the weather was bad, but I don't care none about weather. I'll go out anytime I get the chance.

Mrs. Tubber took me to the library so I could get me a library card, so I could take books home to read. She showed me how to fill out the card: you put your name and address. Then she give it to the lady at the desk. The lady said, "You could take out two books today."

I told her, "Oh, thank you."

Mrs. Tubber left me there so she could go shopping. It was a big library, it was a good-smelling library, smelled of books. I seen the sign, said "Childrens' Books" and I went over to that side of the room. The desk lady called out to me real loud, "Those are the childrens' books." I guess she thought I was making a mistake 'cause I'm a grown-up. And that did make me feel funny even though there wasn't many people in there to hear it. I said, "Oh, that's okay, I don't mind," and I just kept going, didn't know what else to do. I can't read grown-up books too good.

I set down on the floor and pulled out books and looked at them, put them back on the shelf, pulled out more books. I never seen so many books in all my life; there was much more books than Mrs. Knopf has in the school library. Too many books. I didn't know how to choose just two, I could of took fifty with me.

When Mrs. Tubber come back, I was still setting on the floor. Got a pile of books on the floor, too, and I was reading a book about Helen Keller. The book told that Helen Keller was a girl who was deaf and blind, then they learned her to talk with language on the fingers. She had tampers, too. It put me in mind of me a little bit.

Mrs. Tubber said, "Winifred, you been here an hour. Hurry up and pick out what you want and put the rest of them books back on the shelf. I got groceries in the car."

So I choosed the Helen Keller book and I just grab up the book that was on top of the pile, it was about Noah and the Ark, but when I try to stand up I couldn't 'cause my feets was sleeping. From too much setting on top of them. So

Mrs. Tubber had to put most of the books back for me, Mrs. Tubber took the books I choosed to the desk lady to tell her these was the books Winifred wanted. I had to just set there and rub my feets until they was feeling okay enough to walk.

When we come out, it wasn't raining no more. We stop at a house so Mrs. Tubber could buy eggs, but I didn't even want to get out of the car, didn't even care to see the chickens. I was too busy reading about Helen Keller.

Next day I ask Mrs. Tubber, "Don't you people go to church here?" 'Cause it was Sunday. But she said no.

I read, wrote a letter to Mrs. Knopf, then I ask Mrs. Tubber could I go for a walk by myself. Maude was taking a nap. She said, well, okay, don't get lost.

I walked a different way, not the grocery store way, I walked to the fields. And kept going into the woods. The trees was in their autumn colors already; you think God threw paint all over everything. A teeny little squirrel was setting by a tree looking at me. I hollered, "Hi, squirrel!" I heard a train whistle. It sounded like the train was crying, a lonely sound. The wind was making my hair blow.

I felt free. Free as a bird.

45

When Mrs. Handelman come, we set together on the big porch. She asked me how was I doing. I told her, "Good!" I told her, "I think the outside world is wonderful! I been to town three times already, I got a library card, even take walks every day all by myself. You wanna take a walk with me?"

She said, "Sure," so we walk up the street and I show her

the grocery store, also showed her the brown and black dog. I petted him, Mrs. Handelman petted him, then we went back to the house. Mrs. Handelman said, "Did Miriam call?"

"Miriam? She don't know where I even am."

"Yes, she does, 'cause I talked to her on the phone, give her your number. She said she was gonna call you up."

"Well, I sure hope she does, I sure hope she'll come see me."

Mrs. Handelman, before she left, she ask me was I having any problems. That's the main thing social workers are for: help you fix your problems.

I told her, "Yes, I got a problem. Nobody here goes to church, so how am I suppose to go?"

She said, "I'll talk to Mrs. Tubber, see what we could work out." She did, too. She got Mrs. Tubber to talk to some people across the street, tell them to take me to church with them every Sunday.

And the next week Miriam called me up, said how do I like this place, said she was gonna try and come see me soon. She said, "Do you need anything, like a jacket or a coat?" I said yes, I sure could use a coat, 'cause it was starting to get chilly and the institution only give me summer stuff and one sweater.

Caroline and the other ladies in my room went and told Mrs. Tubber I didn't take no baths and Mrs. Tubber got mad. Said, "How come you didn't take no baths, and you been here close to two weeks?"

I said, "Nobody told me to. Anyway, I don't care for baths, I care for showers."

"Then take a shower, Winifred. Look at your nails, look at your hair."

I took a shower, then I washed my hair. The sink wasn't working too good, you could tell it was a real old sink, and when I was done washing my hair the sink was all plugged up and water was coming all over the floor.

Grace and Althea come up the stairs. Grace said, "Look at that!" Some people come out of their rooms to look at that and Althea said, "What did you stick down that sink?"

"Nothing, I didn't stick nothing."

We was standing out in the hall by Laura's room so our feets wouldn't be wet. Laura was a teeny old lady, got a teeny room, she played with dolls. Never come out of that room. Someone carried up her food on a tray every day. She was always in there taking care of them dolls.

Mrs. Tubber come upstairs with one of the men, see if they could fix the sink. I told her, "Don't blame me, I don't even know nothing about this place. I'm only a new kid here." She had to go back downstairs, call the plumber.

Every time I ask Mrs. Tubber if me and Maude could go to town alone, she would growl, she would say, "Oh God." She was nice, but sometimes she liked to growl.

I told her, "I like taking walks, I like going to the grocery store, but now I wanna go to town. We could take the bus. I know where it stops."

"You never been on a bus alone."

"So? I could learn, couldn't I?"

"Wait until Saturday, I'll take you to the library."

I didn't think that was fair. That's not how you're suppose to treat someone who's out in freedom now. I asked her again when she was out raking leafs, she was looking more friendly. "Mrs. Tubber, why can't we go to town alone? We're not in jail, we're not in no institution no more."

"Well, Winifred, I feel that maybe you girls won't come back."

"I wouldn't run away from here."

"I don't know, I don't trust you yet. Maybe you're gonna meet someone, maybe something's gonna happen."

"Don't worry about men, Mrs. Tubber, if I wanted a man so bad I could of got one before I come here. But I'm not man-crazy."

She kept on raking, then when all the leafs was piled up together she said, "Okay. I'm gonna trust you, see how you do."

I hollered, "Oh, boy!" jumped right in that big pile of leafs. Leafs all over me, even in my hair. Mrs. Tubber had to laugh.

Next morning I was all in a dither, put my nicest dress on, put my hair up in a ponytail, wash my face two times. I had six dollars saved up; I put it in the pocket of my sweater, and Mrs. Tubber wrote down the phone number of the house so we could call if we had problems. She walked us to the bus stop, told me, "Slow down, slow down," 'cause I was skipping and running all the way.

I seen the bus first, seen it coming up the street. I said, "Maude, here comes the bus!" Almost knocked Maude down, couldn't wait to get on it. She told me, "Look where you're going, will you?"

The seats was nice, big and soft. We set in front near to the driver and I told him, "We're going to town, that's where we want to get off." He said "Okay," and he started singing. Sang "Jimmy Crack Corn" all the way into town and I sang, too, 'cause I knew that song. But Maude just set and looked out the window. She's not the singing kind of girl.

It wasn't a long ride, but it sure was the most fun ride I ever took. I was sorry when we got to town, sorry when it come time to get off the bus. The driver showed us where to wait for the bus when we was ready to go home, right across the street from the school. I told him, "Thanks, I had a real good time."

First we went to the toy store. There was dolls and toy bears, toy pussycats and toy puppy dogs, there was games and books and paints and a wonderful doll house full of rooms and got furniture in there, too. I told Maude, "Oh, I sure like to live in a house like that."

Maude buyed a box of crayons, then we went to the store

that sold clothes such as dresses, blouses, and slacks, and we looked at the clothes, but we didn't touch nothing. We went to the drugstore and I bought me a lipstick, a pretty pink lipstick. Mrs. Tubber didn't care if I wore lipstick, it was okay by her. It was such a joy to go wherever we choosed to go, whatever store we wanted to go in, and didn't have to ask nobody. Just pick out which store, then go in it.

"Lunchtime!" I told Maude.

We went to a restaurant, we set at a table near the window so we could watch the people going by outside. I helped Maude read the menu. When the waitress come over I ordered, told her all that we wanted and done it right, too. Told her, "Maude wants a turkey sandwich and chocolate milk, I want a chicken sandwich and chocolate milk." Chicken is my favorite 'cause it was Gladys's favorite. The waitress wrote down everything I said on her tablet and I felt so important. Like a big deal. Just like all the other people. Oh, I didn't even feel like I was a nervous girl or nothing!

My lunch cost a dollar thirty and Maude's lunch cost a dollar thirty-five. I paid for Maude 'cause I had more money than she did, and I left a tip for the waitress, too. Fifteen cents. I told Maude, "Let's go out more often!"

We went back to the bus stop over by the school and when the bus come we told the driver—it was a different driver—where to leave us off. And he done it, too.

I was so proud. I was learning how to travel.

46

For a long time after I come to Tubber's, I'm waking up all the mornings thinking I'm still in the institution. Thinking institution things, like I gotta hurry get in line for a shower, then it's time for roll call, then go to the cafeteria. And I open my eyes and see them purple flowers on the wall, see them windows with cranks for opening. Sometimes I could smell the breakfast Miss Patsy is cooking downstairs.

Then I know I'm not in the institution no more, then I know I'm in the outside world, and I get to feeling good from my feets up to my head.

On a Sunday after church Miriam come to see me. She said, "Oh, Winnie, what a nice place."

"I'll show you around," I told her, and I showed her the dining room where I eat, showed her the living room which had a rug on the floor, showed her the kitchen, took her upstairs and showed her my room.

"That's my bed and that's my dresser," I told her, "and outside them windows is apple trees."

"You sure got a pretty room," she said.

She got a big bag with her and she dumped it on my bed. Clothes. For me. A brown coat, a couple sweaters and skirts. Even a white purse.

"Try them on," Miriam said. So I put on the coat first. It was a little too short on me, even in the arms, but not too bad. The sweaters and skirts was a little small, too, but I really did like them. One of the skirts was red and green, like stripes.

"Did you buy all this stuff for me?"

"No, they was my stuff, but I don't need them no more. I thought you could use them."

"Oh, I sure could. Thanks."

I showed Miriam the picture of Thomas. It was in my dresser, I didn't want the other people to see it so I kept it in my dresser under my bloomers.

"Who's this?"

"My boyfriend. His name is Thomas, he's from Kortland. Do you like him?"

"Well, if he's okay with you, he's okay with me."

I took Miriam to Maude's room so I could introduce them together. I said, "Miriam, this here's my friend

Maude." And I told Maude, "This here's my sister, Miriam." Maude was laying on her bed drawing pictures. Didn't pay us no mind, just kept on drawing pictures. She's like that, she's nice but she's strange. One time she'll talk to you, the next time she won't talk to you. She comes from an institution, too.

I even give Miriam a peep at Laura, opened up the door a teeny bit so she could look in. Laura was setting on a chair brushing the hair on one of her dolls. Her whole bed was full of dolls, little heads poking out of the covers. They looked to me to be asleep. I told Miriam, "Them dolls sure do keep her busy."

I wanted to show Miriam the grocery store, too, where I go almost every day, but she said, "If I'm gonna take you out to lunch we better go now, Winnie."

I wore the brown coat to lunch, even though it wasn't cold, and I brung the white purse.

Mrs. Handelman had a talk with Mrs. Tubber about a job for me 'cause I was having a problem with getting bored. At the institution there was always something for me to do, but at Tubber's there wasn't always something for me to do. And it was quiet all the time, nothing happening. I like quiet but not that kind of quiet. I like another kind of quiet. If I ask Mrs. Tubber, "What should I do?" she'd tell me, "Read a magazine." So I'd read a magazine, then I'd go tell her, "Well, I'm done. Now what should I do? And it's a long time till supper, too." She'd tell me, "Winifred, you're bothering me to death."

So Mrs. Handelman and Mrs. Tubber worked out that I would have a job and my job was gonna be to help Miss Patsy do the supper every night. Four o'clock every day I gotta report to the kitchen, except Monday when Miss Patsy don't come in. Monday the cleaning lady stays and does supper.

I ask Mrs. Handelman, "Do I get paid?"

She said, "No, you don't get paid 'cause you get your money from the State."

I start my job that day. Miss Patsy was fixing hamburgers and mash potatoes, she told me to set on the stool by the sink and peel the potatoes. Give me a peeler and a whole pail of potatoes. Showed me how to peel. It took some practice, make that peeler do what I want it to, but I did get all the skin off them potatoes. Miss Patsy praised me, said I catched on fast.

After supper I was laying on my bed reading the Bible, which I try to read mostly every night before I go to sleep. The Bible helps me quite a lot, I have faith in the Bible. And I heard Mrs. Tubber calling me, calling, "Winifred, Winifred" so I went to the stairs and she said, "Come down 'cause your sister is on the phone." I went down in my nightie, didn't have no robe to put on, and she told me to pick up the phone in the kitchen.

"Miriam! Are you coming to see me again?"

"I can't this week, Willy's real sick with the flu. I just called to tell you Daddy Kruller died."

"My daddy died?"

"He died last month. Only I just found out about it to-day, so I thought I better call you."

"Why did he die?"

"He was old, Winnie, and his heart was real bad."

"Did my mother die too?"

"No. She's the one called me up."

"Well, tell her I said hello."

I went back up to my room. I was sorry my daddy died, but I didn't feel real bad like when Gladys died. I didn't see him in such a long time, I could hardly even think what he looked like.

47

Me and Maude went to the movies. Mrs. Tubber dropped us off when she went shopping, and we give her our promise to take the bus right away home soon as the movie was done. 'Cause when you're in freedom, you gotta be trustworthy.

We paid, got our tickets, but I got mad when the man inside tried to take my ticket away from me. Told him, "I don't have to give it to you." Maude said yes, I did, Maude said that's how you prove to the man that you paid. She was at the movies before so she knew. But why do they tear it up and give you a little piece back?

It smelled yummy in the movies. Popcorn. Me and Maude had to get us some of that popcorn so we could eat it while we was watching the movie. The popcorn was warm and got butter on it, too.

I seen lots of movies in the Assembly Hall, but they never showed nothing like this. It was about a man and a lady—they was both more beautiful than the other—and they was in love together. But the bad part was they was already married to other people. So they had to go and sneak about it, meet at nighttime. Once they met in a garden, a flower garden. They done a lot of kissing. That's mostly what they done when they met with each other, kissed and kissed. And I don't know what all else. Maude, when the kissing parts come on, she put her face in her hands, said, "Oh no, oh no." She wouldn't look. She didn't like the movie, too much kissing for her. But I cried at the end 'cause the man got killed, the man died.

That movie give me a funny dream. I remember that dream real well 'cause I never had one like it before. It was about Thomas, me and Thomas. And we was beautiful. The dream was in a place, not the institution, not Tubber's—but a little like Tubber's only it had all them flowers. And we was in them flowers kissing like anything. That made me feel strange. I never kissed before, not Thomas or nobody. It's against the rules. If they catch you kissing, you can't go to the dances no more.

But when I woke up with that dream I sure did want to go right back to sleep again.

Every day but Monday I help Miss Patsy do the supper work. Peel potatoes, sometimes I tear up pea pods to get out the little peas stuck in there, also Miss Patsy showed me how to make salad. You need lettuce, tomatoes, and cucumbers, you cut them all up, put them in the little salad bowls. Learned to make fruit salad, too, you use fruit for that. One job I didn't like was cutting up onions. That always brings the tears to my eyes. I was glad to be working in the kitchen, though. I knew I was getting good training.

Sundays I go to church with the Deckers, Mr. and Mrs. Decker that live across the street. On Sundays, when I come back, many a times there is visitors, families coming to see the old people. Even with little kids. I feel shy when them people come, also feel bad that no one is coming to see me. I know if Gladys didn't die, she would be always coming to see me. Gladys was more faithful than Miriam, no one could be as faithful as Gladys was. Bless her little soul.

Once Maude's mother come. She was nice-looking, not too old, dressed up pretty, too. Didn't look nothing like Maude. They set in the living room and she was trying to get Maude to talk to her, saying things to Maude and waiting for Maude to say things back to her. But Maude just set there holding the cookies and candy her mother brung, wouldn't say nothing, wouldn't even look at her. You could tell she didn't like her mother, you could tell she wanted her mother to go away. Maude shouldn't do like that, she should feel lucky she got a mother; she should be proud she got a mother who comes to see her.

After her mother left, Maude went up to her room with

her goodies and ate them, ate them all herself. Didn't even share with her friends.

I ask Mrs. Handelman if she could call up my mother. When Mrs. Handelman called up Miriam, Miriam come to see me. I thought maybe if she called up my mother, that could make my mother come to see me. But she never come. Never even wrote me. Could be she's sick, or maybe she's just forgettable.

But I did get a real nice letter from Thomas. I liked it that people could write to me and I could write to people, tell them anything I want, and Mrs. Tubber didn't read it. That's how they do in the institution. They read every darn letter you write, read every darn letter you get before they give it to you. By the time you get your mail, it's stale news. I hate that. I think it's snoopy.

Thomas in his letter asked me to send him Miriam's address so he could write a card to her, tell that he's Winifred's boyfriend. Also said he's lonely for me, said he hopes someday we could be together again.

I went to the grocery store and bought me some Scotch tape. I got Thomas's picture out of my drawer and I sticked it up on the wall with tape. Marie started hollering that I was gonna mark up the walls. I told her, "Well, how am I suppose to hang it up, then?"

"Get a frame, put it on your dresser like I do." When Caroline come up to get her medicine, Marie told her, "Look what Winifred done."

"You can't do that," Caroline said. "You'll tear up the wall paper."

I told them, "It's not your house, it's Mrs. Tubber's house, so you can't tell me what to do."

Marie said, "But it's our room."

"So what? It's my room too."

Marie had to march right downstairs to Mrs. Tubber to tattle on me. Got Mrs. Tubber in her room, she was laying down with one of her sick headaches and she was angry to be bothered. She come upstairs, told me to take the picture down right now 'cause it was gonna ruin the wall paper.

Also the ladies tattled on me about being messy, said I left my clothes all over the floor. That wasn't true. Sometimes I left them on my bed and they drop down to the floor, but is that my fault? Mrs. Tubber blamed me again, said I gotta do better habits.

I hate tattletales.

I wrote a letter to Mrs. Knopf, told her I miss her, told her I can't trust nobody at Tubber's 'cause everyone's always ratting on me what I do.

On the first day of snowing, I dress up real warm with my brown coat and Maude's mittens, Mrs. Tubber found me some boots, and I go for a walk in the snow. It was cold but I didn't care, I found it such a joy to walk wherever I wish to walk. The snow come down all over the ground, all over me. I stuck out my tongue to taste it.

The woods was turning white. Autumn colors all gone and now the winter color. I went smushing through the woods 'cause best of all I love to walk in the woods, love to feel that there is nobody but me and God's work.

After awhile I was getting wet and cold. I start to go back, then I hear that train whistle again. I wanted to find that train, get on it, go wherever it takes me. Anyplace.

48

I went to the library, looked for books about places such as New York, Hawaii, and China. I wanted to learn all about them different places, so if I go traveling I could pick out wherever to go.

First I read about New York. Got the Empire State Building, the zoo, tall buildings. The McKennas been there. But I don't know if I would want to go, I heard it wasn't so nice anymore. They got gangsters now. I think New York was nicer when it first come out.

I found a big book with pictures of Hawaii. Boy, is it ever beautiful in Hawaii. No gangsters there. You could eat coconuts, you could put flowers in your hair, wear them cute little skirts, lay around the beach all day, and soon as you get to feeling hot, you just jump in the water. Bare feets—don't need your shoes in Hawaii. That's the life for me!

One day in the morning time I took the bus into town. Didn't tell no one where I was going, didn't even tell Maude. I had a plan to get me a job, a real job. Then I would have lots of money to save up for traveling. I could get me an easy job to start off with, then harder jobs when I learn more training. And maybe someday, when I was done traveling, I could be a nurse. In the white dress, in the little cap, a helping nurse.

When I got my job, then I would tell Mrs. Tubber and Mrs. Handelman. Would they ever be surprised. They would say, "Well, look what Winifred done. She went out and got herself a real job."

I went to the restaurant where me and Maude had lunch. There was a lady in there, a waitress, and she was busy giving all the people their food, so I stood by the door. Then, when she wasn't busy, I went over and told her, "I don't want to order nothing, I just want to get a job here."

She said, "You gotta see the boss. He's in back, in the kitchen."

I was real nervous. Like, did I look okay? I got on my nicest stuff, the red and green skirt and the red sweater and the brown coat, ponytail on my head real neat.

There was a man in the kitchen cooking stuff in a big pot. Lunch food, I guess. It sure smelled good. I ask him, "Are you the boss?"

He said, "Yes. What do you want?"

"A job, I want a job. I thought maybe I'll work in a restaurant. I could peel your potatoes, I could mash your potatoes, I could make jello, I could cut up your salad for you."

He put down the spoon, the big spoon he was stirring with, he said, "Where you working now?"

"I help Miss Patsy in the kitchen. At Tubber's, that's where I live. Tubber's Nursing Home. That's not real close, but I do know how to go on a bus."

"I know where Tubber's is. How old are you, anyway?"

"What do you think, I'm almost thirty-two. So I'm old enough now to work in a real job, old enough now to work in a restaurant."

He started stirring again, turned around and put his back at me, told me, "Sorry, we don't need no help."

"Well, maybe you don't think I could do things, but you're wrong. I'm not dumb, I'm smart. I know about kitchens and I know about fixing food."

He told me, "Lady, I told you I don't need no help, just get out of here now." Stirring, stirring, stirring.

I went outside, stood in front of the restaurant. I knew I done it wrong, knew I done something wrong. He thought I was peculiar.

Then I turn around and seen him, that boss, he was standing by the window with the waitress. They was looking out at me.

I walked very fast away from that place.

When I come back to Tubber's, there was an ambulance in the driveway. Mrs. Tubber told me, "Go in the living room and stay there." She forgot to even ask where I been.

I said, "But why?"

"Never mind why, just go."

The old people was in the living room, too, most of them standing by the door like waiting to be let out. Maude was the only one watching television. I ask her, "What happened?"

"I don't know. Somebody's sick."

I ask Caroline and Grace who was sick, but they didn't know. They was all trying to figure out who was here and who wasn't here. Some of the people go up for naps after lunch, some go for walks if it's not too cold, and Bridey went to the beauty parlor with her daughter. Sam said maybe it was Laura who was sick.

Then we heard people coming down the stairs loud—the ambulance people, I guess—heard them go out the door, and the old people rush right out of the living room looking for Mrs. Tubber. In a little while there come a scream.

I told Maude, "I gotta see what's going on out there." Maude stayed there looking at the television. She don't appear to care much about nothing.

Everyone was in the kitchen and Caroline was setting at the table with Mrs. Tubber and Winston. Got her head down on the table and making noises. I think she was crying.

I ask Sam, "Why is Caroline crying?"

He said, "Marie died."

"Marie died?"

"Poor thing," the cleaning lady said, "she just laid down to take a nap, never got up again."

"Marie died in our room?" I ask her. She said yes. I went back to the living room, set down with Maude by the television.

All day I was afraid to go up to my room, even to put away my coat. I thought maybe the ambulance people didn't take Marie, maybe they left her still in bed, dead. Mrs. Tubber was talking on the phone until almost supper time, had to make a lot of calls about Marie being dead. I thought maybe when she was done I could ask her did they take Marie or didn't they take Marie? I waited by her office room a long time. When she wasn't on the phone no more, I went in.

She said, "Why the heck was you hanging around out there, Winifred?"

I said, "Never mind."

★   ★   ★

I stayed in the living room. Nobody was playing cards tonight, but a few people did watch television. Caroline just set on a chair holding onto her cane, didn't talk to nobody. After awhile she put on her sweater and went up to bed, then the others started to go up. I was tired, I had a long day, town and everything. But I watched television until the news was on, then Mrs. Tubber come in, said, "Winifred, everyone's in bed, what are you doing down here?"

I told her, "I'm going, I'm going. Don't rush me."

I went up the stairs. I tippytoed down the hall. The little light was on, but I was scared to go in my room. So real slow I peep in. I thought, if Marie's still in there I'm going back downstairs and I don't give a darn what Mrs. Tubber says.

But her bed was empty. No Marie there, no sheets there, no blankets there, even the pillow was gone. Like nobody slept in that bed ever before.

I tippytoed in. Althea was in bed and by the window was Caroline, just standing there looking out at the dark. I set down on my bed, took off my shoes and socks, my skirt and sweater, my underclothes, sticked them under my bed. Took my nightie out from under my pillow and put it on. I got into bed and pulled the covers all the way up, far as they could go.

On Thanksgiving we had a turkey. Mrs. Tubber and Miss Patsy and me was all in the kitchen buzzing around, doing the cooking, and some of the old ladies helped, too. Me and Bridey done the stuffing—she showed me how—and that was fun.

Some of the old people went home to their families, some didn't go home. Miriam said I couldn't come to her for Thanksgiving 'cause they was going to Wanda's, said maybe I could come for Christmas. But I didn't go for Christmas 'cause they went to Florida. That was okay by me, though. I didn't wanna go to Miriam's house, I didn't wanna have to see Willy.

A new lady come to take Marie's place in her bed. Her name was Celeste and she was grumpy.

49

The toy store had a sign in the window. It said, "Christmas Help Wanted." Maude and me went in. I told the lady, "I could help for Christmas."

She said, "What do you mean?"

"The sign. Christmas help. I could help with the toys, 'cause I need a job."

"Are you working now?"

"Sure I am. At Tubber's Nursing Home. In the kitchen."

"Did you ever work at a store before?"

"No, but I could learn to do it."

"We need someone who worked at a store before, we need someone who could run a cash register. So I don't think this is the right kind of job for you."

"Well, what do you think would be the right kind of job for me?"

She smiled at me friendly, said, "That's a question I can't answer."

Maude and me looked around the store a little, all them pretty toys. We petted the soft animals. When we left I told the lady, "Bye-bye, thank you."

She said, "Good luck."

When we got outside, I told Maude, "I'll never get me a job, I'll never get me lots of money to save up. I'll never go to Hawaii."

She said, "Maybe you just gotta keep looking."

On the way to the bus stop I went into the bakery.

Didn't have no sign in the window, but I like bakeries, I like the way bakeries smell. There was a man behind the counter, must be the baker, he had a white apron like Miss Patsy wears. He was selling a pie to a lady. When the lady left, I told the baker, "Could I get a job here? I don't know how to run a cash register, but I could learn. I really like bakeries."

He said, "Sorry, we don't need nobody."

"Not even to help with Christmas?"

"Nope."

Maude bought a bag of cookies. She give me one and we ate them on the bus going home. I ask Maude, "Do you think that baker thought I was peculiar? Do you think that's why he wouldn't give me a job?"

She told me, "You're not peculiar."

"Well, thanks, I'm glad you said that."

Next time Mrs. Tubber took me to the library, I went to a bunch of stores, six or seven, but nobody would give me a job. Some of the people wasn't even too nice about it, neither. I run back to the library in time to meet Mrs. Tubber. She said, "How come you didn't get no books today?" I told her, "I didn't want to." I was feeling cross. Anyway, I didn't always like to go to the library now. Sometimes kids would stare at me when I was there. Like they was thinking, what's wrong with her, why can't she read grown-up books? I didn't like when that happened, it made me ashamed. Once I went to the grown-up books just to show them kids I wasn't retarded. I looked and looked a long time, but couldn't find nothing I could read. So I just pick out two fat books, go marching past them kids carrying them important-looking books. Couldn't read them when I got them home, but I sure was proud to be taking them out.

Every night Winston left his false teeths in the bathroom. The others with false teeths, I guess they put them in their rooms when they went to bed. But Winston's teeths was always floating in a glass full of water on the windowsill, smiling at me.

I told Maude, "You dare me to hide them?"

She said, "Where?"

"I'll find a place."

When everyone was asleep I sneak into the bathroom, take the teeths out of the glass and wrap them in a towel, put the towel of teeths in my top drawer.

Next morning you could hear Winston hollering for his teeths, yelling, "I'm gonna find the person who took my teeths! They'll be sorry!" Sam told him, "It was Winifred, believe me, Winston, it was Winifred." They figured it out right away. Who else would do a thing like that?

I had to stay in my room all day, Mrs. Tubber made me, but at least I had a little fun, made a little excitement in that place.

Then more troubles. I threw a hairbrush at Althea. It was her hairbrush—I couldn't find where mine got to —and when she come in and catched me using hers, she yelled. Told me, "Put my hairbrush down and don't never touch my stuff again." I was gonna put it back, I was gonna be nice, but then she said, "Sometimes I think you don't have no brains in your head." When people say things like that to you, about no brains in the head, it gets you very disturbed. So I threw the hairbrush, hit Althea in the leg.

Mrs. Tubber had a talk with me in her office. I told her I couldn't help getting disturbed 'cause my nerves was starting to get bad again. When my nerves is bad, it makes it real hard for me to behave right, when my nerves is bad, every little thing gets underneath my skin. And anyway, Althea shouldn't never of said what she said.

Mrs. Tubber ask me was I taking my nerves pills every day. I said yes. She said, "Well, I don't care what Althea said to you. I'm still gonna have to tell Mrs. Handelman about this, that you threw a hairbrush, that you hit some-body."

Had to stay in my room all day again, too.

Next time Mrs. Handelman come she took me to a doctor, a private doctor. She said maybe my old pills wasn't work-ing for me no more, said could be the doctor had better pills for me to take.

He was nice, the doctor was, the type that laughs and jokes with you. He give me an exam, he weighed me. He talked to me and I told him how my nerves get the best of me, then I get disturbed, I get all worked up.

He said, "Well, I know just the right kind of pills for you. What's your favorite color?"

"Pink!"

"Oh, you're so lucky, 'cause the kind of pills I'm gonna give you is pink, and they're much better than your old pills." My old pills was orange. He give me a prescription and Mrs. Handelman took me to the drugstore to get the pills. And they was pink. I had to pay for the pills out of the money the State give me.

When we come back to Tubber's, Mrs. Decker was there. She was waiting on me. She wanted to meet Mrs. Han-delman, talk to her about my communion. Father Bryan, where we go to church, said I could make my first commu-nion in May if I went to catechism classes. And if Mrs. Handelman could get hold of my baptismal certificate. I was proud that I could make my first communion, I was thrilled, but I didn't know if I was baptized or if I wasn't baptized, so Mrs. Decker wanted to ask Mrs. Handelman. Mrs. Handelman said she didn't know neither, said she'd look in my files soon as she got the chance.

For Christmas Sam and Lester hung a big wreath on the door, and there was a little Christmas tree on the television, but it wasn't a real one. Nobody cared to make decorations, nobody cared to sing the carols, nobody cared to do nothing special. I did go to midnight Mass with the Deckers, and on Christmas we ate turkey, but that's all. Wasn't even no presents for me, except Miriam sent me five dollars from Florida. I got Maude a Christmas present, a box of candy, but she forgot to buy me a present. Maude forgets things a lot.

There was snow on the ground, it was a white Christmas. I went for a walk, untied the black and brown dog from the fence, took him with me. I could tell he wasn't having no merry Christmas neither. I let him loose in the field and we run, we run through the snow. I chase him, then he chase me. I tripped while I was running, on a rock or something, fell down in the snow. You should of seen that dog. He jump on me, he lick my face, my ears, wouldn't let me up, and I'm laughing so hard I would of fell if I wasn't down already. When I got up I was all wet and snowy, my hair was wet, got snow down my boots and even in my mouth. And still laughing. That was the best part of my Christmas Day, that was joy, me and the dog having good times together.

But when we come back to the dog's house, the man was out in the yard, the man that owned the dog. He was waiting on me. He tied up the dog again, took me back to Tubber's to tell what I done.

Mrs. Tubber said, "Shame on you, Winifred, taking that man's dog away and you didn't even ask."

The man told me, "Stay out of my yard, you hear?"

I said, "I hear."

On the day after Christmas, me and Maude went to the movies again, went to see *Cinderella*. It wasn't in real, it was in cartoon, and I loved it. Cinderella is so beautiful. That was always one of my favorite stories from the time I was little; I use to have that book at home. But the movie was better than the book. The singing, the mices, the pretty clothes Cinderella wore, the handsome prince, the Fairy

Godmother. I wish I could have a Fairy Godmother doing all that stuff for me. Fairy Godmothers are wonderful. They're a little like social workers, only magic.

The pink pills was working. That doctor was a good doctor, I could tell, 'cause the pink pills was better than the orange pills. I could sleep at night without jumping in my sleep, didn't have so many bad dreams, felt relaxed even to my fingers and toes.

And I was trying very hard to change from worse to better. It wasn't easy, I knew some of the people didn't like me. Althea and Winston wouldn't even talk to me no more. But still I was trying. I smile at people. If I was setting in Lester's chair by the television and he tell me to give him back his chair, I wouldn't say, "No, I was here first," I would get up, go set someplace else, not give him a hard time.

Mrs. Handelman was sick a couple weeks with the flu and I didn't see her, but she did call me. Said how was I doing with the pills. I told her good, I was doing real good. Then she ask to speak to Mrs. Tubber. I know she wanted to find out if I was behaving okay or if I wasn't behaving okay, but I wasn't worried about what Mrs. Tubber would tell her. I knew I didn't do nothing wrong for awhile.

When she got over the flu, she come to see me. We set in the kitchen and Mrs. Tubber made her a nice hot cup of coffee. Mrs. Handelman took something out of her pocketbook, a big envelope, opened up the envelope and took out a big piece of paper. Said, "I found your baptismal certificate for Mrs. Decker, Winifred, and I want you to look at it." She give it to me, I read what it said. It wasn't my name on there.

"This isn't about me," I said.

"Yes, it is."

Mrs. Tubber took the certificate, she read it. "Gwynna Sprockett? Who's Gwynna Sprockett?"

"That's Winifred," Mrs. Handelman said. Didn't look

like she was joking, neither. "I think when Mrs. Kruller took you to the institution when you was little and told them your name was 'Winnie,' the clerk or someone put down 'Winifred.' Must be the clerk thought 'Winnie' was short for 'Winifred.'"

"'Winnie' isn't short for 'Winifred?'"

"Sometimes it could be, but turns out your 'Winnie' is short for 'Gwynna.'"

"And they changed her name on her?" Mrs. Tubber said. "Well, I never heard of such a thing."

Mrs. Handelman said, "I have."

I was feeling real mixed up. "You mean my mother, my real mother, named me 'Gwynna' and a clerk named me 'Winifred?'"

"Looks that way to me," Mrs. Handelman said.

I told Mrs. Handelman I didn't think that was fair. She said she didn't think it was fair, neither.

But I guess there wasn't nothing I could do about it. I guess it was too late to change it back to what it should of been. Guess I was stuck being 'Winifred.'

50

I went to all the stores on the library side of the street. Even the paint store. Nobody had a job to give me. I was getting sick of trying, I was telling myself, "Oh, what's the use?"

It was way past my lunchtime. I didn't want to go to that restaurant, the restaurant with that boss, so I went to the little place by the library where you gotta set at the counter 'cause they don't have no tables. Ordered me toast and root beer. I couldn't get more food 'cause I had to save my money for the bus.

There was a little girl and a mommy setting next to me at

the counter. The mommy was trying to get the little girl to eat her hamburger. The little girl kept saying, "No, I want a hot dog." She had braids like I use to have, she was cute, a real normal kid. I love to see real normal kids.

I give her a big smile, she give me a big smile. I told her, "If you don't want that hamburger you could give it to me. I'll eat it."

Little girl said, "Oh, mommy, the lady will eat it, then you get me a hot dog."

The mommy said, "Eat your hamburger, the lady's just joking with you."

"No, I'm not joking," I told her. "I'm hungry. If your little daughter don't want that hamburger, I sure be happy to eat it for her. Why don't you get her a hot dog?"

The mommy got up, took the little girl off the stool, took the hamburger, carried them down to the other end of the counter. Come back to get her plate and the sodas and went back and set down with the little girl. Told her, "Shush up now and eat."

I finished my toast, I paid my check, I went to the lady and told her, "I'm not peculiar!" But she made like she didn't even hear me.

There wasn't no one in the library when I come in, so I went to the children's books. I was setting on the floor reading a funny book, I was laughing. And I look up and there was two girls setting at one of them little tables, must of come in while I was busy reading. I seen them in the library before, they was some of the kids who liked to stare at me. They was staring at me again.

I said, "What are you kids staring at? I'm laughing 'cause this is a funny book. Did you ever read this book?" They started laughing, too. Covered their mouths with their hands so I couldn't see. But I could hear them.

I said, "Why are you laughing? What's so darn funny, anyway?" They wouldn't answer, they was laughing too hard. At me.

I hollered, "Shut up, you kids, shut up, you got no rights to be laughing at another person!" And they shut up. I guess I scared them. But there was some other people in the library and they was looking at me, too. Even the desk lady.

I bust into tears. Set there on the floor holding my book and cried. And everybody watched me. Then I got up and run right out of that library.

Behind the school, in the play yard, there wasn't no one to watch me. I wipe the snow off one of the swings, set down. I cried, I rocked the swing, I cried some more. My nose was running, had to keep wiping it on my coat sleeves 'cause I didn't have no hanky.

After a long time I started to walk.

Near the school was a house with a big hill. There was a whole bunch of kids out there with sleds. They was wearing snowsuits of all bright colors such as red, blue, and green, and they was going down that hill on them sleds fast as anything I ever seen before. Like flying. It looked to me like a picture in a story book. I watched them for awhile, but I stood behind a tree so they couldn't see me.

I walked some more. I knew the way to go, I walked the way the bus goes. It took a long time, took a lot of walking, and when I got to Tubber's, it was dark. I could tell it was way past four o'clock. I knew Miss Patsy was gonna be mad, I knew Mrs. Tubber was gonna be mad, I was afraid to go in the house. But I was cold and tired. Hungry, too.

Mrs. Tubber, when she seen me, she nearly yelled my head off. Said she went into town looking for me, said she was getting ready to call the police. She told me to come in her office.

I said, "I'm cold, I'm hungry."

"Well, I'll make you some tea, warm you up. After we talk, you could go get a sandwich 'cause you missed supper."

We set in her office, I had my tea in there, and she said, "Now you better tell me what happened, Winifred."

I said, "Nothing. I went to a restaurant, I went to the library, then I walked home."

"You walked all the way home? Why did you do that? Didn't you have no bus money?"

"I had money. I just didn't want to go on the bus, didn't want to see nobody."

"Winifred, I got a phone call today," she told me. "The lady from the flower store. She said you been in there three times asking for a job, said you told her you work here. Said she tells you she don't need no help, but you keep coming back bothering her."

"I wasn't bothering her, I was polite."

"And she told me you been next door to the drugstore a couple times, bothering them for a job, too. Winifred, why was you looking for a job?"

I started to cry again, I don't know why, but I just start crying. Mrs. Tubber had to take my tea away, I was getting tears in it. She said, "What are you crying about?"

"Please, Mrs. Tubber, I don't want to talk, I don't want no sandwich, just only want to go to bed now."

"Okay," she said. "Go to bed. We'll talk tomorrow."

Mrs. Handelman come the next day and it wasn't even Wednesday. We set in Mrs. Tubber's office, without Mrs. Tubber, so we could talk private. I told her, "I know why you come. You come 'cause I got in troubles."

She said, "Well, Mrs. Tubber told me what happened yesterday. And she told me you been going into stores in town, bothering people to give you a job."

"I wasn't bothering."

"This morning she called the lady at the library, see if you really was there yesterday or if you wasn't there. The lady told her you was, the lady told her you was yelling at some little girls and scared them half to death."

"They laughed at me."

"Winifred, I want you to think about something, I want

you to think about going back to the institution. Maybe you wasn't ready to get out yet."

"You think I'm too dumb, you think I'm retarded, you think I'm not smart enough to live in freedom!"

Mrs. Handelman said, "Calm down, calm down," and when I was calm down she said, "I'm not saying you're not smart enough. You just been living in the institution so long you're not use to living on the outside. You gotta try real real hard to get use to it, and maybe you're not ready enough to try real real hard."

"So you're taking me back, right?"

"No. I'm gonna let you think about it. You could stay at Tubber's if you want, but no more going in town. You gotta stay right here by the house."

"Not even the grocery store?"

"Nope. You could only go places with Mrs. Tubber. And church. She don't trust you no more. How could she?"

I woke up in the middle of the night 'cause someone was shaking me. It scared me, it did, I thought maybe it was a robber. But it was Althea. She told me, "Can't you even shut up when you're sleeping?"

"Well, what did I do?"

"You been yelling half the night, that's all, keeping everybody up."

"I can't help it. Sometimes that's how I do."

Caroline and Celeste was awake, too, all grumping that they was sick of me and sick of my big mouth. I got out of bed, I told them, "Leave me alone, just everybody leave me alone!" I could hear them still grumping about me while I was going downstairs.

It was dark down there, all the lights out. I put on the little lamp in the living room, I set down in Lester's chair. My hands was shaking, my teeths was chatting.

I felt like I didn't even belong to this place. They should of sent me to a better place. Or maybe back to the institution. Maybe that was the place I belong to.

*   *   *

In the morning time, I couldn't get up. Felt sick. Mrs. Tubber come upstairs to take my temperature, said, "You don't have no temperature, so why don't you get up?"

"I can't. I don't feel good."

"Mrs. Decker's coming soon, take you to church. You don't want to miss catechism class, do you?"

"I can't help it, Mrs. Tubber, I feel sick."

I stayed in bed three days, just only wanted to sleep. Sometimes Maude brung me up my food, sometimes Miss Patsy. Miss Patsy was real nice. When I told her I'm sick, she said, "Yes, I could see, you don't look good." She believed me. But that jerk Mrs. Tubber didn't, kept coming up to take my temperature every night, telling me I'm not sick. And Wednesday morning she come into my room, told me, "Okay, Winifred, get up, get dressed."

"No. I'm sick."

"I'm tired of hearing about you're sick. Mrs. Handelman's coming today, you could tell her about it. Now get out of that bed."

I got out of bed, I got dressed and put my coat on. Didn't even brush my hair or brush my teeths. When Mrs. Tubber seen me come down with my coat on, she said, "Where do you think you're going?"

"Don't worry, I'm not going to town, I'm just going out on the porch. What do you care if I'm sick?"

I was setting out on the porch crying when Mrs. Handelman come. She said, "Winifred, what's wrong?"

"I'm sick, I don't feel good, and my nerves is bad. And Mrs. Tubber don't even believe me. I don't wanna stay here no more. Please take me back to the institution before something's gonna happen to me."

Mrs. Handelman took me inside, told me to go upstairs and lay down. She called Mr. Buckholz at the institution. She told him Winifred don't feel so good, Winifred wants to come back.

He said, well, bring her back.

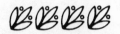

WINTER–
SPRING
1964

51

"How much longer, Mrs. Handelman, how much longer?"

"Winifred, that's the tenth time you asked me that question."

"But are we almost there?"

"Not yet. You sure are feeling better, aren't you?" I was feeling better. I was feeling a lot better soon as we left Tubber's. Could be it wasn't the flu, could be it was homesick.

"It's gonna get dark soon," I told Mrs. Handelman.

"Don't worry, you'll be there in time for your supper."

We drove some more, then I could tell we was near the town. I seen the little stores which are at the end of town near the institution. Then a little more driving and guess what, the gates!

"We're here, we're here!"

We drive through the gates, up the driveway past the Office Building and the Psychology Department and the office workers' parking lot, then we turn and turn again and there was Meadow. Mrs. Handelman parked in front of the building in the circle. You could do that if you're a social worker, they'll let you leave your car there.

I jump out before she was even finished stopping the car and up the steps I run. First person I seen was Mrs. Gaynor, she was in the front hall buttoning up the coat for one of the girls. The girl was trying to get away from having her coat buttoned.

"Well, look who's here," Mrs. Gaynor said.

"Hi, Mrs. Gaynor." I could smell the building smells, smelled just right to me. Friendly.

Mrs. Handelman come in carrying my suitcase, said, "Winifred, wait up."

"I gotta go see everybody, say hello."

"They gone to the cafeteria, honey," Mrs. Gaynor said. Mrs. Handelman told me to go on over and get my supper, she had to talk to Mrs. Demerest.

Boy, was it noisy in the cafeteria, I forgot how noisy. Girls talking and laughing and yelling. First person I seen was Kissy. She was setting at a table by the door eating all by herself, except for her baby doll. And Ruby Rose was at the table next to her, with Billie and Amelia and Antonia, the table where we always set. Right away Ruby Rose seen me, hollered, "Look, it's Winifred!"

"Hi, hi," I told them.

"I thought you wasn't coming back!" she said.

"I didn't like it there, and anyway I wasn't feeling so good."

"I knew she was coming back. I told you so," Billie said.

Antonia said, "You got a new coat."

They was all eating, it was meat loaf for supper. I went and got a tray, got a fork and spoon, stood in line behind some girls from Spruce. Miss Dobie seen me, she use to be a night attendant at Meadow, then they sent her to Spruce. She come over to say hello to me while I was waiting in line. Said, oh, it's good to see you, stuff like that, told me I was looking skinny. I did, I did look skinny, Miss Dobie was right. Then two of the Spruce girls start banging each other with trays and Miss Dobie had to go break it up, make them girls behave theirselfs.

One of the cooks give me a plate with a big piece of meat loaf, also put peas and mash potatoes on my plate. I went back, set next to Antonia, gobbled up that food. The institution has good food, better food than Tubber's got.

"Franny got out," Billie told me. "Only she didn't come back."

"Franny got out? Where to?"

"Nursing home. My social worker says I'm gonna get out, too. Maybe in the summertime, maybe in the fall. And I'm not coming back here, neither."

I told Billie, "You wait. You think it's gonna be peaches and beans when you get out, but it isn't. Them nursing homes is full of grumpy old people. When you get out you're gonna be bored, just plain bored."

"No I won't. 'Cause when I get out, me and Aldo is gonna get together," she said, and she and Amelia start laughing so hard they almost fell off their chairs.

I ate up all my food, cleaned my plate, finished the meat loaf that Ruby Rose left, too.

When we come back to Meadow, Mrs. Handelman was gone, but she left my suitcase in Mrs. Demerest's office. I took it upstairs, give it to one of the attendants so she could unpack me. I didn't get my same bed back, somebody else had it. They give me a different bed, but I liked it 'cause it was closer to the windows. My old bed wasn't closer to the windows.

Then I went down to find Ruby Rose and there she was in the Day Room with some of the others, they was watching a movie on television. It was a funny movie. When the man in the bathtub stood up, he had his shorts on. Real crazy. We was all laughing and joking and one of the girls was talking back to the people in the television, saying silly things. Everybody having a fine time. I felt very joyful.

52

Mrs. Knopf give me my job back. Said she rather have me work for her than somebody else work for her. 'Cause I'm so trustworthy.

Mrs. Knopf said could be it was all for the best that I come back to the institution. Like, if anybody's in a place a long, long time, it might be real hard for the person to get use to living in another place, a different place. Same thing Mrs. Handelman said.

"So sometimes it's better for a person to stay where she's use to it," Mrs. Knopf told me, "where she fits in to it."

I think she was right, too, when she said that. 'Cause the institution raised me up, the institution is my home. More friends here for me to talk to.

"When you was out there, did you see my mother?" Ruby Rose ask me.

I told her no.

"You didn't see her? You didn't see her no place?"

"Nope."

"Well, when you was out there, did you go to town?"

"Sure I did. And went to the library, went to restaurants, even the movies."

"Oooh, you're lucky."

"Nothing so great about town," I told her. "When you go to town all the time, you could get tired of going to town. You could even get bored of it."

"I wouldn't get bored of it."

That just shows how smart she is. But it's not her fault, she wasn't in the outside world like I was. I know about the outside world now, know about the outside people, too. But I thought, well, maybe I better not tell her.

★ ★ ★

When it come to be Mrs. Knopf's birthday, I give her a card I made. I cut out pictures of flowers from a magazine, paste them on the card. I know she loves flowers. Inside the card I wrote, "You may not be my mother, but anyway I respect you and I wish you was my mother." I had to ask Mrs. Krause how to spell "respect," the other words I could spell all by myself.

Mrs. Knopf loved that card, said it was real nice of me to do a thing like that, make a card. I told her, "Well, I don't have no mother to give her a birthday card and you don't have no children to give you a birthday card. So that's why I thought it would be a good thing!"

"Don't you send no cards to your foster mother?"

"No, I don't send her nothing. Never hear from her and I hope I never do. Can't be bothered."

We was eating our lunch in the teachers' office. Mrs. Knopf always brings her lunch, and on days I'm working for her she packs me lunch, too, so I don't have to go to the cafeteria. Sometimes she even brings stuff from her garden when things is growing. Such as green peppers, tomatoes sliced up. I like it that I can eat my lunch with Mrs. Knopf.

"You know, Winifred, I still got your book that you was writing."

"You do?"

"Well, I told you I was gonna hold it for you. You want it back now?"

"Okay."

We clean up, throwed out our bags and napkins and stuff, then she goes digging through her drawers, found my book. Told me, "I was gonna give this back to you, anyway, 'cause in June I'm gonna retire."

"Retire? You won't work here no more?"

"I been here thirty years. I'm ready for a rest."

"But what will you do, what are you gonna do if you're not coming here all the days?"

"Gonna sell my house. Gonna move in with my brother and help him out. He can't walk much now." Mrs. Knopf use to have a husband, then he died, so Mrs. Knopf had to live all alone by herself.

"I won't see you?"

"Oh, sure you will. I'll be around, I'll come to visit. Work with the other teachers sometimes."

"Well, that's okay. Long as I still get to see you."

I was dancing with some boy and Ruby Rose come over, ask me to go to the bathroom with her. When we come out, I walk smack into Thomas.

He said, "Winifred!"

"Thomas, I didn't know you was here!"

He didn't look good. There was years in his face. He grab up my hands, said, "I thought you wasn't never coming back."

"Well, I come back last month."

We went over to one of the tables, we set down. I felt funny, you could say I felt shy of him. I was thinking of the dream I had about him when I was at Tubber's. I wonder can people sometimes tell when you dream about them?

"Do you still like me?" he ask.

"Sure I do," I told him. "I won't dance with nobody but you."

They was playing a slow song, a pretty song, on the Victrola. Me and Thomas danced together. There was lots of people dancing, we kept bumping and banging into them. Thomas don't dance real good, but that's okay. I don't dance real good neither.

"I'm getting awful old, Winifred."

"Yes, I know."

He was hugging me so tight while we was dancing and he stepped on my big toe hard, said, "'Scuse me for stepping on your feets all the time." I look up and seen his eyes full of tears. The tears was going down his face and his face was all over wet and shiny.

Two of the Kortland attendants come over, ask me, "What's wrong with him?"

I told them, "He's not crying 'cause he's sad, he's crying 'cause he's happy to see me. I'm his girl."

We took Thomas out to the hall where it wasn't crowded, where it wasn't noisy, and one of the attendants got him a napkin so he could wipe off his face, blow his nose. And all the time he was hugging and hugging me, just didn't want to leave go.

The attendant who got the napkin, she told the other attendant, "We could leave them alone out here. They are two sweethearts, but they don't do nothing wrong, no kissing or nothing. Let them hug, they're happy to see each other."

After they left, we set there awhile. I had to go get Thomas another napkin, the first one was wet.

"You know, Winifred, I saved up my money and I got me a radio. And I listen to my radio every day."

"That's nice, Thomas." I helped him wipe his eyes. I got him a drink of water.

"You won't go away again, will you?"

"I don't think so. It's up to my social worker, I guess."

He put his arms around me again. "Oh, Winifred, I wish I could get married with you."

53

Mrs. McKenna come by to see me, she was down visiting Jeannie. I don't know how she knew I was back, but she did. I was real glad to see her. She ask me did I want to come with her to visit Jeannie. I said sure, sure I did.

Same smell, same low-grades yelling and carrying on. But I didn't even care so much, didn't even mind so much. You could say after I been away so long and come back again, everything in the institution was looking okay to me. Even Forest.

Jeannie just got done being sick. Mrs. McKenna told me first she catched the flu, then she catched bronchitis. Poor little Jeannie, she looked like an old skinny dog, she did. But she smiled at me.

I told Mrs. McKenna, "I know you can't get down here a whole lot, but you don't need to worry about Jeannie now I'm back. I'll start looking after her again like I use to look after her."

And soon as Mrs. McKenna left, right over to the canteen I run. Buyed a pack of cookies and a little thing of milk. Then I go back to Forest, put the milk in a paper cup and bust up the cookies and put the cookies in the milk. That's how you have to do for girls who got no teeths. They can't chew up cookies.

I held the cup for Jeannie and she drunk it, drunk up every little bit. She liked it. I told the attendant, "I don't mind spending my money on Jeannie, I'm happy to do it. 'Cause she needs them cookies more than I do, she needs to get back her weight."

Mrs. Knopf kept all the time asking me was I working on my book again, I kept all the time telling her no, too busy. So then she said, "Well, I wasn't gonna tell you this, but while you was away I showed your book, what you wrote already, to a couple doctors in the Psychology Department. And they thought it was real interesting stuff."

"They did?"

"And they told me if you ever finish it, they might put it in a doctor's magazine. Publish it."

"Publish it?" I almost popped from proud. "For everyone to read?"

"For doctors to read."

"Not my family?"

"You could send it to them. If it gets published."

"What if it don't get published?"

"Then I could type it up for you real nice on my typewriter and you could send it to them anyway."

So I start writing again. Only I wasn't gonna let them just put it in a magazine. I was gonna make them put it in a real book, like Pearl Buck's book. To be in the library. To show people I'm intelligent upstairs, show people I got something up there instead of nothing. Brains. To write books and stuff.

Mrs. Knopf said it's very hard to get books published, said don't put your heart on it or you'll be disappointed. But I did put my heart on it.

On the days I work for Mrs. Knopf I bring my book, set at the desk and write while I'm waiting for the phone to ring, while I'm waiting to take the messages. I get lots of writing done there. The phone don't ring much. In the nights I set in the bathroom to write 'cause they leave the lights on in there.

Mrs. Demerest had to tell me, "Winifred, I don't care how much you write in the daytime, but when it comes night you gotta put your book in my office and go to sleep. You're getting rings underneath your eyes from not enough sleeping."

"And headaches," I told her. "I'm getting sick headaches."

"Well, that's from too much writing."

It was from too much attendants, too. They was teasing me and that was getting me very disturbed. Dr. Kravitz give me back my old orange pills for my nerves, no more pink pills, and they was helping until the attendants started dogging me. Saying my head was getting swelled up from writing.

And Mrs. Krause told me, "You better stop acting like a big shot, Winifred. All of us is getting plain sick of hearing you boasting and showing yourself off. Think you're something special, don't you?"

I told her, "I sure do, I sure do think I'm special. I'm writing a book. I bet you can't write a book!"

"Maybe I can and maybe I can't, none of your business if

I could write a book. Just shut up your big mouth or I'm gonna report you."

I cussed her out, she went right down and told Mrs. Demerest, and I had to stay in the building all day. They wouldn't even let me go to Mrs. Knopf.

I told Mrs. Krause, "Goody, goody, I'm glad I gotta stay in the building. Now I could work on my book all day long."

The low-grades was down in the Day Room and the music lady was playing the Victrola for them. Some was in wheeling chairs, some was on the floor, the ones with good muscles was setting up by theirselfs in chairs. The music lady played "Oh, Susannah" and "The Yellow Rose of Texas," played them both over two times.

One of the low-grades was sleeping and a couple looked like they didn't want no part of this world. But most was having a fine time. I feel sorry for the low-grades. They could never have a normal life, too far gone. But they could feel happiness sometimes. I know. When they hear that music they laugh, and the smart ones even clap hands. They love music. It fills their little hearts. I brung a chair over to Jeannie, I took her little hands and helped her clap. She didn't know what the heck we was doing, but you could tell she was having fun.

When the music lady left, the attendants put the low-grades out in the sunshine. But they let Jeannie stay in 'cause I brung haircurlers to curl up Jeannie's hair. The attendants said, "Jeannie could stay in 'cause Winifred is gonna fix up her hair for her."

I took her into the bathroom, put a little water on her hair, rolled up her hair on the curlers. She set real still and didn't fret, she knew I was making her pretty. Jeannie's an easy child to handle. Some low-grades will kick and bite and scratch you, even pull off the glasses you got on your face. Then the attendants have to smack them. But Jeannie don't do none of them things, Jeannie has a sweet personality. Anyway, I wouldn't let none of them attendants smack her and they know it, too.

Mrs. McKenna, when she was carrying Jeannie, got measles; she told me that's why Jeannie is retarded. So it's not Jeannie's fault. She couldn't help it. None of the low-grades could help it, that's why we gotta try to be kind to them. They didn't ask God to make them low-grades. How could they?

After I got the curlers in, I let her stay outside until her hair was mostly dried up. And when I comb it out all the attendants come buzzing around to fuss over Jeannie, tell me what a good job I done. I told them, "Well, maybe I should get me a job in a beauty parlor!"

Then I took Jeannie for a walk to show her off. I got special permission to take her for walks. I pushed her all the way over to the Assembly Hall and back. I know Jeannie is retarded but I'm not ashamed of her. I'm proud of her.

54

In the days, in the warming-up days, I write outside. I set under a tree on the front lawn. It's pretty there, it's peaceful there for writing.

I tell everyone I'm writing a book. The other girls say, "Oh no, you're not." So I say, "Wanna bet?" and I show them my book, show them how much I wrote already. Then they know how smart I am, then they can't call me retarded.

If I get my book published, everyone will read it, everyone will know how smart I am. And Willy will 'gratulate me.

I was setting out there writing when the fire happened. I seen the smoke coming up behind the boiler house. Lots of other girls was out on the lawn too, but they was all walking and talking and waving at cars. I'm the only one seen the smoke.

I run across the lawn, I run around the boiler house. The smoke was coming from a truck, from inside a truck that was setting out behind the building. Boy, did I ever use my head. I flew for help. Right into the boiler house I run and I call to Jake Johnson—he works there—I call, "Jake, Jake!"

He said, "What's the matter, kid?"

"Smoke's coming out of that truck!"

He run to the window and looked out, said, "Oh my God, stay there," and he went and called the office, told them to hurry up send police and fire engines. Then we go outside and wait. He told me, "Keep back, keep back, 'cause the gas in the truck might explode."

People was starting to come around, see what was all that smoking for. There was some attendants, too. They was shooing away the girls, telling them, "Get out of here, go away." But I wouldn't go. I told them, "I'm not moving, I'm not moving an inch, and you can't make me. 'Cause I'm the one seen the fire first, I'm the one reported it to Jake Johnson."

Two big fire engines come. The firemen jump off, they had to get an axe to bust open the window and then they squirt some stuff into the truck. Not water, it was white stuff. They had to pull the seats out of the truck, throw them on the ground, put water on them. Then the fire was all out.

Mr. Buckholz was there, too—he's dead now—and Jake Johnson said, "This is the kid," and he pointed at me, said, "This is the kid who told me about the fire."

Mr. Buckholz said, "Where was you going, Winifred?"

So I told him, about that I was on the front lawn and seen the smoke, nobody else seen the smoke but me, and I run to the boiler house and seen it was coming from the truck and I thought, "I got to get some help!" And I told him, "I

wasn't thinking about myself, Mr. Buckholz, I was thinking about the institution. What would happen if the gas ex-
ploded? What would happen? All them girls and cripple
children in the institution, they could of got hurt."

He had me down in the office the next day. They was all
buzzing, asking me questions and writing down what I said.
I told them I'm not sure what started the fire, but I think it
was too much heat. You gotta leave the windows open a
little bit so the air could get in, but Jake Johnson had them
all tightened-up closed. And they showed me some cigarettes, they found them near the truck, they ask me do I
smoke cigarettes. I said, "Sometimes, but they're not
mine." I said, "I have my own." Mr. Buckholz sent someone with me to Meadow so I could show them what kind of
cigarettes I got. I don't use the kind with filters, I use the
same kind as Dr. Kravitz.

They wanted everybody's matches, too. The supervisors
of the buildings made all the girls line up and give them
their matches. But they didn't get mine. I hid mine.

Mr. Buckholz thanked me, he told me, "You done a
good thing, Winifred. I bet you saved the whole institution."

That was my very biggest thrill. Saving the institution from
getting all burned up. It was all over the institution, too,
what I done. Was I ever proud! But the girls was dogging
me again, teasing and teasing, saying I was boasting and
showing off.

"Well, what would you do?" I told them. "Just leave the
institution go? Not me! I think of all the other girls besides
me living here."

"Then you should of left it burn up," Billie said.

"We'd all get out of here," Edith hollered. "We'd have
freedom!" And everyone yelled, "Freedom!" Everyone
clapped hands.

"Oh, you all think freedom's so wonderful," I told them.
"That proves how much you know. You wasn't in it. All

freedom is a nursing home with old people and got false teeths, and when you go to town everyone thinks you're peculiar! That's all freedom is!"

Mrs. Potts come in, said, "You girls, shush up and get into bed. It's after nine o'clock."

We all got in our beds. Since I come back from Tubber's, I'm in the next bed to Kissy. Her baby doll was already tucked in, she puts it to sleep early. Mrs. Potts turned off the lights, Mrs. Potts went out. But you could talk, you're allowed to talk until nine-thirty if you're quiet, if you don't be silly.

Ruby Rose come tippytoeing over, set down on my bed, said, "Do you know what my mother looks like? I can't remember her face too good."

"I can't remember her face neither," I said.

"Well, then, how do you know you didn't see her when you was out?"

"I don't know. Maybe I did."

"It's better to be in the institution, isn't it? Isn't this a real good place to live?"

I told her, "No."

"No? But you said. You're always saying it."

"It's only better for us," I told her. "'Cause we're use to it here. Now shut up, Ruby Rose, I wanna get me some sleep."

Anyway, I think some day I'm gonna get another chance to get out. Mrs. Handelman said she'd see about it. When I'm ready enough to try real, real hard.

EPILOGUE

Five years after Winnie's return to the institution, she was placed in another nursing home. Though she had the intelligence to function in the community and was clearly capable of holding down simple jobs, it was just too late for her, after nearly a lifetime of incarceration, to make the massive adjustment required to live outside institution walls. The only alternative available to her, a nursing home—where she had no peer group and there were no vocational or recreational programs to suit her special needs—undermined her chances of success even more. A year after her release, she begged to be returned to the safety and familiarity of institution life. This time she was placed in another institution, one that was very near her sister Miriam's town. And this is where she remained until her death in 1976, at the age of forty-four, of uterine cancer.

In the course of researching this book I interviewed a number of people connected with the State and with both institutions. I found that there was a question, a very big question, about whether Winnie had really been clinically retarded. In the opinions of those who'd worked most closely with her (including Eva Handelman, her social worker for eight years), her retardation was functional: that is, acquired after birth. In other words, in the opinions of the people who knew her best, Winnie was a classic example of an extremely deprived childhood. Winnie used to say that if her parents hadn't died when she was a baby, she'd probably never have ended up in an institution. It seems very likely that she was right.

The times were against her, too. Today's relatively new community-based group homes for the mentally retarded, still in experimental stages in some places, are already proving to be an effective alternative to institutionalization for the mildly and moderately retarded. Group-home residents are able to move on to independent living with a higher success rate than that of their institutionalized counterparts, and even those who remain in the group homes permanently lead far better lives in a pleasant, homelike atmosphere. Winnie would have been an ideal candidate for group-home placement. Unfortunately, no such system existed then.

Winnie Sprockett left a precious legacy: her voice. Through it she gives a rare insight into the world of the mentally retarded, a world most of us can't even begin to imagine. Through it she speaks for the nearly six million mentally retarded men, women, and children in the United States. Hopefully, she helps us to understand. And to care.

'Gratulations, Winnie.